COACHING
in MEDICAL
EDUCATION

The AMA MedEd Innovation Series

The Master Adaptive Learner
Edited by William Cutrer, Martin Pusic, Larry Gruppen, Maya M. Hammoud, and Sally Santen

Value-Added Roles for Medical Students
Edited by Jed Gonzalo, Maya M. Hammoud, and Gregory W. Schneider

Coaching in Medical Education
Edited by Maya M. Hammoud, Nicole M. Deiorio, Margaret Moore, and Margaret Wolff

COACHING in MEDICAL EDUCATION

The AMA MedEd Innovation Series

MAYA M. HAMMOUD, MD, MBA
University of Michigan Medical School
American Medical Association

NICOLE M. DEIORIO, MD
Virginia Commonwealth University School of Medicine

MARGARET MOORE, MBA
Institute of Coaching, McLean Hospital

MARGARET WOLFF, MD, MHPE
University of Michigan Medical School

ELSEVIER

Elsevier

1600 John F. Kennedy Blvd.
Ste 1800
Philadelphia, PA 19103-2899

COACHING IN MEDICAL EDUCATION,
FIRST EDITION

ISBN: 978-0-323-84726-1

Notice

Practitioners and researchers must always rely on their own experience and knowledge in evaluating and using any information, methods, compounds or experiments described herein. Because of rapid advances in the medical sciences, in particular, independent verification of diagnoses and drug dosages should be made. To the fullest extent of the law, no responsibility is assumed by Elsevier, authors, editors or contributors for any injury and/or damage to persons or property as a matter of products liability, negligence or otherwise, or from any use or operation of any methods, products, instructions, or ideas contained in the material herein.

Publisher: Elyse O'Grady
Senior Content Development Specialist: Jennifer Pierce
Publishing Services Manager: Catherine Jackson
Senior Project Manager: John Casey
Design Direction: Patrick Ferguson

Working together
to grow libraries in
developing countries

www.elsevier.com • www.bookaid.org

Printed in India

9 8 7 6 5 4 3

CONTRIBUTORS

Atul Agarwal, MD
Assistant Professor of Clinical Radiology and Imaging
  Sciences
Indiana University School of Medicine
Indianapolis, Indiana
Chapter 8

J. Aaron Allgood, DO
Chair of Clinical Science Education
A.T. Still University School of Osteopathic Medicine in
  Arizona
Mesa, Arizona
Chapter 5

Indira Bhavsar-Burke, MD, MHPE
Chief Fellow, Gastroenterology and Hepatology
Indiana University School of Medicine
Indianapolis, Indiana
Chapter 7

Rebecca Blankenburg, MD, MPH
Clinical Professor and Associate Chair of Education,
  Pediatrics
Stanford University School of Medicine
Stanford, California
Chapter 10

William B. Cutrer, MD, MEd
Associate Dean for Undergraduate Medical Education
Vanderbilt University School of Medicine
Nashville, Tennessee
Chapter 2

Nicole M. Deiorio, MD
Associate Dean, Student Affairs, Professor, Emergency
  Medicine
Virginia Commonwealth University School of Medicine
Richmond, Virginia
Chapter 1

Basim Dubaybo, MD
Vice Dean of Faculty Affairs and Professional Development
Wayne State University School of Medicine
Detroit, Michigan
Chapter 11

Donna Elliott, MD, EdD
Professor of Pediatrics and Medical Education
Vice Dean for Medical Education
Chair, Department of Medical Education
Keck School of Medicine of the University of Southern
  California
Los Angeles, California
Chapter 9

Michele A. Favreau, PhD, MSEd
Professor Medical Education
Sam Houston State University College of Medicine
Huntsville, Texas
Chapter 12

Matthew Fitz, MD, MSc
Vice Chair for Faculty Development, Department of
  Medicine
Stritch School of Medicine, Loyola University Medical Center
Maywood, Illinois
Chapter 2

Micaela Godzich, MD
Associate Professor of Family and Community Medicine
Director of the Academic Coaching Program, School of
  Medicine
Associate Residency Program Director
UC Davis School of Medicine
Sacramento, California
Chapter 9

Larry Gruppen, PhD
Professor
University of Michigan Medical School
Ann Arbor, Michigan
Chapter 2

Michael A. Haight, MD, MHA
Clinical Professor, Pediatrics
Pediatric Gastroenterology
University of California, San Francisco
San Francisco, California
Chapter 12

Maya M. Hammoud, MD, MBA
Professor, Obstetrics and Gynecology
University of Michigan Medical School
Senior Adviser, Medical Education Innovation
American Medical Association
Ann Arbor, Michigan
Chapters 1 and 7

Antwione Haywood, PhD, MED
Associate Director for Diversity, Equity, and Inclusion, IU
    Simon Comprehensive Cancer Center
Assistant Professor of Clinical Radiation Oncology
Assistant Dean for Student Affairs, Medical Student
    Education
Indiana University School of Medicine
Indianapolis, Indiana
Chapter 9

Jean E. Klig, MD
Director, PEM Student Programs
Massachusetts General Hospital
Director, Clinical Learning Coaching Program
Assistant Professor of Emergency Medicine and Pediatrics
Harvard Medical School
Boston, Massachusetts
Chapter 12

Tai Lockspeiser, MD, MHPE
Assistant Dean of Medical Education–Assessment,
    Evaluation, and Outcomes
University of Colorado Anschutz Medical Campus
Aurora, Colorado
Chapter 2

Kimberly D. Lomis, MD
Vice President, Undergraduate Medical Education
    Innovations
American Medical Association
Chicago, Illinois
Chapters 2, 7, and 8

Andrea Marmor, MD, MSEd
Clinical Professor of Pediatrics
San Francisco General Hospital
UCSF School of Medicine
San Francisco, California
Chapter 10

Hilit F. Mechaber, MD
Senior Associate Dean for Student Affairs
Associate Professor of Clinical Medicine
University of Miami Miller School of Medicine
Miami, Florida
Chapter 9

Mark Meyer, MD
Professor, Family Medicine
Senior Associate Dean, Student Affairs
University of Kansas School of Medicine
Kansas City, Kansas
Chapter 8

Jennifer R. Miller, MD
Associate Professor of Pediatrics
Penn State Health, Milton S. Hershey Medical Center
Hershey, Pennsylvania
Chapter 9

Amy Miller Juve, Med, EdD
Associate Professor
Vice Chair, Education, Department of Anesthesiology and
    Perioperative Medicine
Professional Development and Program Improvement
    Specialist
Graduate Medical Education
Oregon Health & Science University
Portland, Oregon
Chapter 6

Margaret Moore, MBA
Co-Founder and Chair
Institute of Coaching, McLean Hospital
Belmont, Massachusetts
Chapters 1 and 3

Ronda Mourad, MD
Associate Professor
Case Western Reserve University School of Medicine
Associate Clerkship Director for Internal Medicine
Louis Stokes Cleveland VA Medical Center
Cleveland, Ohio
Chapter 6

Binata Mukherjee, MD, MBA
Assistant Dean, Faculty and Professional Development
College of Medicine/Mitchell College of Business
University of South Alabama
Mobile, Alabama
Chapter 8

Elza Mylona, PhD, MBA
Professor, Internal Medicine
Vice Provost for Faculty Affairs and Institutional Effectiveness
Eastern Virginia Medical School
Norfolk, Virginia
Chapter 11

Kendra Parekh, MD, MHPE
Assistant Dean for Undergraduate Medical Education
Associate Professor of Emergency Medicine
Vanderbilt University Medical Center
Nashville, Tennessee
Chapter 4

Kurt Pfeifer, MD
Professor of Medicine
Medical College of Wisconsin
Wauwatosa, Wisconsin
Chapter 5

Archana Pradhan, MD, MPH
Associate Dean for Clinical Education
Associate Professor
Rutgers Robert Wood Johnson Medical School
New Brunswick, New Jersey
Chapter 6

Carrie E. Rassbach, MD, MAEd
Clinical Associate Professor, Pediatrics
Stanford School of Medicine
Stanford, California
Chapter 10

Rishindra M. Reddy, MD
Professor, Section of Thoracic Surgery, Department of Surgery
Chair, University of Michigan-Comprehensive Robotic Surgery Program
Jose Jose Alvarez Research Professor in Thoracic Surgery
University of Michigan Medical School
Ann Arbor, Michigan
Chapter 7

M. Melinda Sanders, MD
Professor of Pathology and Laboratory Medicine
University of Connecticut School of Medicine
New Haven, Connecticut
Chapter 5

Simran Singh, MD
Designated Educational Officer
VA Northeast Ohio Healthcare System
Assistant Dean for Clerkships
Case Western Reserve University School of Medicine
Cleveland, Ohio
Chapter 4

Sherilyn Smith, MD
Professor of Pediatrics
University of Washington School of Medicine
Clinical Skills Learning Specialist
Seattle Children's Hospital
Seattle, Washington
Chapter 4

Christine Thatcher, EdD
Associate Professor of Family Medicine
Associate Dean for Medical Education and Assessment
University of Connecticut School of Medicine
New Haven, Connecticut
Chapter 5

Richard N. Van Eck, PhD
Associate Dean for Teaching and Learning
Monson Endowed Chair for Medical Education
Professor, Population Health
University of North Dakota School of Medicine and Health Sciences
Grand Forks, North Dakota
Chapter 11

Sandrijn M. van Schaik, MD, PhD
Professor of Pediatrics
Baum Family Presidential Chair for Experiential Learning
Vice Chair of Education, Department of Pediatrics
UCSF School of Medicine
San Francisco, California
Chapter 10

Margaret Wolff, MD, MHPE
Associate Professor of Emergency Medicine and Pediatrics
University of Michigan Medical School
Ann Arbor, Michigan
Chapter 1

The American Medical Association's Accelerating Change in Medical Education Consortium is working to create new approaches to health professions training to ultimately improve patient outcomes. Our consortium has produced significant innovations in a number of areas that are being adopted at multiple schools. To assist in the dissemination of these innovations, we are pleased to present a series of books to aid the adoption of these ideas at additional health professions schools and training programs.

The AMA MedEd Innovation Series provides practical guidance for local implementation of the education innovations tested and refined by the AMA consortium. This AMA book on academic coaching is the third in this series. Future subjects will include improving change management for faculty, implementing health systems science education, and incorporating the electronic health record into curricula.

Coaching in Medical Education presents the work of coaching experts inside and outside the AMA consortium who have implemented coaching programs in undergraduate and graduate medical education. As the field of academic coaching continues to grow, we hope you find this book a valuable resource as you initiate or grow an already existing coaching program.

We are pleased to offer this third book in the AMA MedEd Innovation Series and look forward to learning about your experiences in implementing a coaching program at your institution.

Susan E. Skochelak, MD, MPH
Chief Academic Officer
American Medical Association

We are pleased to present *Coaching in Medical Education*.

Coaching is emerging as a framework to provide professional development and assistance to learners in medical education. While long used in the business world, and more recently in patient care and physician circles, coaching is relatively new to the medical education world. Literature is still developing regarding the best coaching practices that will lead to the best outcomes for our learners. To fill this gap, we offer this coaching book. In addition to covering coaching theories, models, and competencies, this book illustrates the important relationship of coaching to the development of the master adaptive learner and offers a practical framework for educators and administrators who are forming and optimizing coaching programs in their own schools.

The first four chapters discuss what coaching is and is not, the relationship to the master adaptive learner, coaching theories, and coaching competencies. Subsequent chapters cover operational aspects of coaching, and the book concludes with a proposed research agenda and discusses the future of coaching. References provide additional reading. Case vignettes are interspersed in each chapter, and the authors have included explicit take-home points. While evidence is cited when available, this book also relies on consensus and best practices from the many coaching programs represented in the American Medical Association Accelerating Change in Medical Education Consortium.

This book focuses most heavily on undergraduate and graduate medical education, though many of the principles discussed span the entire continuum of learners, including continuing medical education. Specific executive coaching for faculty and physicians is beyond the scope of this book, but all health professionals can benefit from the principles covered in herein.

We hope you find this book helpful as you seek to explore and launch coaching programs of your own.

Maya M. Hammoud, MD, MBA
Nicole M. Deiorio, MD
Margaret Moore, MBA
Margaret Wolff, MD, MHPE

ACKNOWLEDGMENTS

The editors and authors of this book would like to thank Sarah Ayala of the American Medical Association (AMA) for her project management. Without her, this book would not exist. We'd like to thank Victoria Stagg Elliott, also of the AMA, for her copyediting and catching our misspellings and misused words. Kevin Heckman of the AMA and project manager of the AMA MedEd Innovation Series gets our gratitude for his support of this book. We give additional thanks to the members of the AMA Accelerating Change in Medical Education Consortium who contributed to this book's creation and to Susan E. Skochelak, MD, MPH, the AMA's group vice president for medical education. Without her leadership, the consortium and, thus, this book would not have been possible.

CONTENTS

COACHING in MEDICAL EDUCATION

Coaching in the Academic Environment

Nicole M. Deiorio, Margaret Wolff, Margaret Moore, and Maya M. Hammoud

LEARNING OBJECTIVES

1. Introduce coaching in medical education and differentiate it from advising, mentoring, and counseling.
2. Explain the rationale for coaching in medical education.
3. Describe the need for this textbook.
4. Briefly introduce each chapter.

CHAPTER OUTLINE

CHAPTER SUMMARY

This chapter introduces coaching in medical education and highlights the rationale for coaching and for this textbook. We describe coaching's application in supporting competency-based medical education and the development of the master adaptive learner. We also provide a brief overview of subsequent chapters to pique the readers' interest.

INTRODUCTION

Coaching has emerged as a promising approach to facilitate learner development and help learners reach their full potential across the medical education continuum.[1] The integration of the coaching approach continues the innovative efforts of medical educators in adapting approaches long utilized in other high-performance professions, such as sports and music.

Whereas coaching has a long history in bolstering corporate and government leadership, helping people improve their businesses and their lives, and supporting health and wellness in the patient care setting, a number of coaching programs have been launched in undergraduate and graduate medical education in the past few years.[2] Interest in coaching

has surged over the past 5 years in part because of the potential role it can play in competency-based medical education, including the integration of coaching skills into clinical skills. To date, coaching in medical education has been used to increase learner well-being, develop technical and nontechnical skills,[3] and facilitate professional identity formation.[2]

For health professionals, the purpose of coaching is the same as for other professionals—to help individuals optimize their professional performance, professional potential, and overall well-being; although, what this looks like varies. By supporting learners in prioritizing their own aspirations, values, and needs, coaches help learners build foundational skills and behaviors for the journey toward a successful career in the continuously evolving field of medicine.[1] The coaching process empowers learners to develop personal visions, identify gaps between their present and ideal states, and create and implement realistic action plans.

DIFFERENTIATING COACHING FROM ADVISING, MENTORING, AND COUNSELING

Coaching is now a unique professional discipline, with specific competencies developed through best-practice processes, as explored in Chapter 4. With a coach's expert

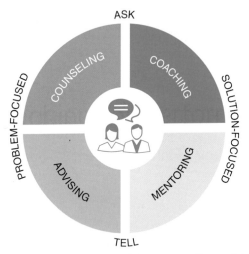

Fig. 1.1 Distinguishing coaching, counseling, advising, and mentoring. (Copyright American Medical Association.)

facilitation, coachees create their own agendas for change, reflecting that they are the best experts in what is ideal for themselves. Two other key tenets of coaching are: (1) asking more than telling, that is, inquiring and facilitating more than advising and educating, and (2) guiding a learner toward personal values-based goals and personalized paths to navigate challenges and reach goals.

In contrast, advising often takes the form of answering questions that the learner brings to the relationship or providing another perspective on a problem. Advisers are expected to be content experts. A skilled coach does not need to be an expert on the topics a learner wants to explore. A mentoring relationship often focuses more on

---

Vignette 1

At a curriculum committee meeting, someone mentions a paper they read on academic coaching and wonders if it would benefit their medical school, especially because the recent Liaison Committee on Medical Education (LCME) site visit found their advising program to be suboptimal.

Thought Questions

1. Consider the traditional faculty roles in your educational program. Which quadrant of the "learner/faculty"–"problem/solution" quadrant do they fall into?
2. How would a coaching program or training faculty to incorporate coaching techniques potentially augment these relationships?

---

cultivating a longer-term professional trajectory. Mentors are also expected to provide not just expertise, but to share their experience in living the path the learner is navigating. Coaching is also distinct from counseling, in which more of the attention is devoted to clarifying, deconstructing, and resolving problems than brainstorming around optimal goals and paths toward goal attainment. Fig. 1.1 illustrates the differences in methods used in these roles, contrasting asking from telling, and a problem-focus from a solution-focus.

Coaching is rewarding for the coach,[4] just as traditional mentoring and advising roles can be. All three provide a close, personal way to have a meaningful influence on a learner's development and growth. No single role is better than another, and different learner situations can call for any of these. Physicians may be most comfortable with the more traditional roles of advising and mentoring in medical education and, as such, may be tempted to default into these modes. Advising and mentoring techniques can potentially undermine the self-determination offered by a coaching relationship, where the coach helps the learner find their own way. Coaches who are also experienced in mentoring and advising are alert to when the empowering role of coaching is called for to improve agency and confidence. They take care in refraining from their prior expert roles as mentors or advisers and minimize giving learners their advice and answers.[5]

RATIONALE FOR THIS TEXTBOOK

With this textbook, we substantially update and expand upon the first American Medical Association *Coaching in Medical Education: A Faculty Handbook*. We cite the most current literature and consensus on best practices on coaching in medical education. We recruited authors for each chapter who are expert coaches, educators, and leaders, most of whom are forming and optimizing coaching programs at their own institutions. Each chapter covers a distinct topic in coaching. References provide future reading. Case vignettes are interspersed in each chapter, and explicit take-home points are highlighted.

COACHING TO SUPPORT COMPETENCY-BASED MEDICAL EDUCATION AND THE DEVELOPMENT OF THE MASTER ADAPTIVE LEARNER

Medical education is embracing competency-based education across the continuum. It is then vital for medical students to become master adaptive learners and "learn how to learn how" to effectively perform a large body of competencies. Coaching skills enable faculty to individualize their approach to supporting each student's individual competency learning needs. Through coaching, faculty can have meaningful relationships with learners that are focused on exploring optimal outcomes, objectively assessing their performance relative to what is optimal, and helping them process feedback positively in service of their own goals for competence and growth. In summary, coaching supports the development of master adaptive learners by inviting medical students to be proactive in their learning processes, assessing their learning, reflecting on feedback, and adjusting their practices to incorporate new learning.

Furthermore, with rapid advances in health care delivery, knowledge, and scientific innovations, physicians are called to integrate ongoing reflection and learning within their practice.[6] Ideally, then, our medical education system would be skilled at cultivating master adaptive learners who use a metacognitive approach to self-regulated learning that leads to the development and demonstration of adaptive expertise in practice beyond medical school.[7] This will ensure future physicians are ready for a continuously changing health care environment, being skilled at learning and adapting to external change while also proactively leading and coaching for positive change.

Over the past two decades, coaching psychology—the science of coaching relationships that are designed to facilitate self-actualization—has evolved rapidly. Dozens of theories and scientific domains are integrated into coaching processes by scholars and practitioners. In this textbook we define coaching and coaching competencies specifically for medical educators, exploring the relevant scientific base of theories and tools. Our goal is to help coaches in medical education integrate an appropriate coaching theory and tool to meet coachees' particular needs and support successful coaching outcomes.

BRIEF CHAPTER OVERVIEWS

We begin in Chapter 2 by offering insight into the intersection of coaching, the environment, and competency-based medical education to support master adaptive learners. In Chapter 3 we define coaching in medical education and explore important theories and models relevant to coaching competencies in medical education, including self-determination, intentional change theory, motivational interviewing, mindfulness, emotional intelligence,

> ### Vignette 2
> A program director notices that at the residents' semiannual evaluation meetings, residents are focused on external motivators such as their in-training examination scores and finding a job after residency, but it has been harder to engage in discussions related to becoming a stronger physician and continuing improvement practices after graduation from residency.
>
> ### Thought Questions
> 1. What strategies can a coach employ to help a coachee tap into internal motivation and focus on longer-term goals?
> 2. How does coaching facilitate goal setting?

positive psychology, goal-setting processes, and cognitive behavioral coaching.

Chapter 4 describes coaching competencies required of an academic coach in medical education, as well as common scenarios and practical advice. Chapter 5 highlights different tools that are utilized in several different coaching models. Applications of coaching—how and when to apply coaching throughout a physician's career—are discussed in Chapter 6. A specific type of coaching—for performance improvement (e.g., surgical skills or communication skills)—is highlighted in Chapter 7, where content experts serve as performance coaches.

The subsequent chapters focus on issues to consider when creating coaching programs in medical education. Building programs with attention to diversity and ethical practices is covered in Chapter 8, and Chapter 9 features detailed examples of successful coaching programs that readers can use as models for their own initiatives. Chapter 10 contains helpful information on creating a strong coach development program.

The textbook ends with content designed to show the value of coaching. In Chapter 11, readers learn how to develop and measure high-level outcomes for their coaching programs. Lastly, Chapter 12 presents available evidence that coaching works, and outlines a research agenda for those who wish to advance the science of coaching in medical education.

We hope this textbook fills a need for those involved in creating coaching programs, informing coaching best practices, and those interested in furthering the science of coaching in the medical education continuum.

TAKE-HOME POINTS

1. Coaching overlaps but differs in significant ways from traditional faculty roles such as advising, mentoring, and counseling.

2. Coaching can be a unique strategy to promote goal and competency attainment, self-actualization, professional identity formation, and a lifelong learning mindset.

REFERENCES

1. Deiorio NM, Carney PA, Kahl LE, et al. Coaching: a new model for academic and career achievement. *Med Educ Online.* 2016;21(1).
2. Wolff M, Hammoud M, Santen S, et al. Coaching in undergraduate medical education: a national survey. *Med Educ Online.* 2019;25(1).
3. Lovell B. What do we know about coaching in medical education? A literature review. *Med Educ.* 2018;52(4):376–390.
4. Brooks JV, Istas K, Barth BE. Becoming a coach: experiences of faculty educators learning to coach medical students. *BMC Medical Education.* 2020;20.
5. Deiorio NM, Foster KA, Santen SA. Coaching a learner in medical education. *Acad Med.* 2021;96(12):1758.
6. Cate OT, Carraccio C. Envisioning a true continuum of competency-based medical education, training, and practice. *Acad Med.* 2019;94(9):1283–1288.
7. Cutrer WB, Miller B, Pusic MV, et al. Fostering the development of master adaptive learners: a conceptual model to guide skill acquisition in medical education. *Acad Med.* 2017;92(1):70–75.

Coaching and the Master Adaptive Learner Model

William B. Cutrer, Tai Lockspeiser, Matthew M. Fitz, Larry Gruppen, and Kimberly D. Lomis

LEARNING OBJECTIVES

1. Describe how the Master Adaptive Learner model supports agility in learning.
2. Articulate the role coaching plays in the individualized pursuit of competency development throughout a career.
3. Identify the impact of institutional culture and the learning environment on the success of coaching and competency development programs.

CHAPTER OUTLINE

CHAPTER SUMMARY

The master adaptive learner is an individual who uses a metacognitive approach to self-regulated learning that leads to the development of adaptive expertise. Coaching serves as a powerful strategy to guide the individual through the master adaptive learning process and should be leveraged to make learners more effective in their learning and development. Central to the success of this model are clearly articulated expectations for the coach to use in supporting the learner, which competency-based medical education provides. Competencies frame the teaching, learning, and assessment methods fundamental to facilitating the learner's progressive development. Additionally, because the learning environment can be such a significant influence on the learning process, we must consider and intentionally shape the environment to optimize learner development.

INTRODUCTION

Physicians and other health care professionals are tasked with delivering high-quality health care while ensuring a positive individual experience of care, improving the health of populations, and reducing per capita costs of that care, all within the context of a rapidly evolving complex system. Traditional approaches to health professions education have not enabled practitioners or the system to accomplish these goals. A new approach is needed to develop practitioners with both the routine expertise needed to effectively and efficiently solve known challenges and the adaptive expertise needed to recognize and address novel challenges. Redesigning health professions education to cultivate master adaptive learners will support ongoing improvements in the performance of both individuals and systems.

In this chapter, we explore the centrality and connectivity of several key medical education topics necessary for expert physicians and systems to deliver high-quality health care. First, we explore the idea of a master adaptive learner who uses a metacognitive approach to self-regulated learning individually or within a group to foster the development of adaptive expertise. Building on the idea of the Master Adaptive Learner (MAL) model, we highlight how the external perspective of a coach can be used to facilitate and amplify this type of learning and expertise development. Next, we turn to the broad themes of competency-based medical education that provide the necessary clarity of expectations and performance data to inform and guide learner engagement with coaching and master adaptive learning. We conclude with exploration of the aspects of the learning environment, the positive and negative influences on coaching and master adaptive learning, and the impact of these contextual factors on the expertise development process.

MASTER ADAPTIVE LEARNER

The MAL model[1] is designed to support the development of adaptive expertise by instilling self-regulated habits that will ultimately position the provider to identify, and respond to, emerging educational needs in a constantly evolving practice environment. Coaches can also leverage the MAL model in early stages of training to help learners meet established expectations of an educational course or program.

MASTER ADAPTIVE LEARNER GEARS

Four gears compose the central elements of the MAL model (Fig. 2.1), representing the four phases of self-regulated learning: Planning, Learning, Assessing, and Adjusting. Iterative learning through these phases provides the foundation that leads to adaptive expertise development.

The gears also mirror the Plan-Do-Study-Act (PDSA) cycle of continuous quality improvement used throughout the health care environment. A master adaptive learner will complete multiple PDSA cycles about themselves as learners, continually deepening their understanding and expertise.

Planning Phase

The planning phase is essential to clearly articulate the gap between what is and what could be or should be. This gap can be related to knowledge, skills, or attitudes and represents an opportunity for improvement. Individuals skilled in gap identification likely recognize many gaps in their own practice within a given day in the classroom or clinical environment; their challenge becomes prioritization among options for learning. Other individuals, less skilled in gap identification, can benefit tremendously from concrete evidence of gaps, such as competency-based performance data, patient outcome data, and external feedback from a peer, supervisor, or coach. When multiple gaps have been identified, it can be overwhelming, especially to more junior learners. The planning process requires a person to intentionally select an opportunity for learning and then search for appropriate learning resources. Many individuals often skip the planning phase, opting to "jump right into actually learning."

Several learner skills will aid in this phase. Questioning is a skill that empowers the individual to look at their current situation (i.e., "what is") and probe whether any gaps exist. The master adaptive learner inquisitively examines multiple perspectives seeking to understand the "what," "how," and "why" of a gap. Prioritizing is an essential skill that allows individuals to elevate one identified gap over others to focus learning efforts. The skills of setting appropriate goals and effectively identifying potential learning resources are effective during the planning phase, setting the stage for the individual to maximize efforts during the subsequent learning phase.

Learning Phase

During the learning phase, individuals spend time and energy critically appraising selected resources and employing strategies for learning. The majority of an individual's effort spent during the learning phase is related to the selection and utilization of learning strategies. Much has been written in both the general education and the medical education literature comparing effective learning strategies that lead to long-term retained comprehension, understanding, and the ability to apply the learning. Unfortunately, trainees and clinicians alike often employ strategies such as rereading, highlighting, and underlining

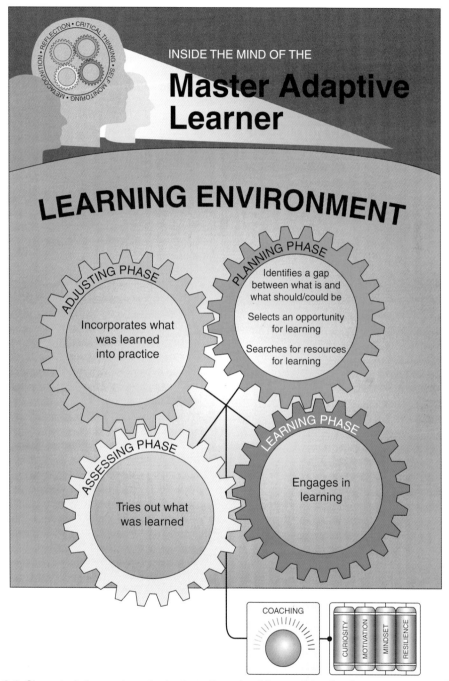

Fig. 2.1 Characteristics and contexts that allow the Master Adaptive Learner process. (From Cutrer WB, Atkinson HG, Friedman E, et al. Exploring the characteristics and context that allow the master adaptive learner to thrive. *Med Teach.* 2018;40[8]:791–796.)

or cramming for exams. These strategies have been repeatedly shown by cognitive science to not support meaningful understanding. Learners would benefit from selecting a learning strategy with sound education science supporting it, such as spaced repetition learning or concept mapping. Such learning strategies require practice and may demand additional investment of time and energy, but they pay learning dividends with continued use. The MAL process itself can be used to allow a learner to identify a gap in their own skills with a selected learning strategy, such as concept mapping, for example, and subsequently allow the individual to plan, learn, assess, and adjust their learning to improve their skills in concept mapping and thus overall learning efficacy. The learning phase is used most effectively when the learner takes advantage of a well-appraised resource and an educationally sound learning strategy to maximize their effort toward addressing a knowledge, skill, or attitude gap identified during the planning phase.

Vignette 1

Stanley is a medical student rotating at the Children's Hospital on his pediatrics core clerkship. Stanley is really excited to be at the Children's Hospital because he is planning for a career in pediatrics. He really wants to perform well on this clerkship and focuses his attention on studying for the subject examination immediately. After obtaining a pediatrics review book, he maps out a plan to read it systematically from cover to cover three times before the subject examination, using a different color highlighter for each pass.

Each student at Stanley's medical school has a personal academic coach with whom they meet periodically throughout the year. Stanley meets with his coach, Jaqueline, halfway through the pediatrics clerkship and expresses frustration that even though he has already read through the review book twice, he can't seem to remember what he has read and really struggles to apply his reading to the individual patients he is caring for on the rotation.

Thought Questions

1. What learning strategies could Jaqueline suggest to enhance Stanley's development as a master adaptive learner?
2. How could Jaqueline provide support and coaching while Stanley tries out new learning strategies?
3. How could Jaqueline prepare Stanley for the additional investment of time and energy that some of the alternative learning strategies will entail?

Assessing Phase

During the assessing phase, learners determine whether they have successfully addressed the gap identified in the planning phase through the use of informed self-assessment. Self-assessment based only on internalized perspectives is notoriously unreliable; informed self-assessment includes seeking external sources of evidence. This information can come in a variety of forms, including scores on knowledge-based examinations, competency-based assessment data, informal feedback, and even patient outcomes. The individual must then interpret and integrate this evidence to respond by either ignoring unhelpful sources, seeking more information in areas that are unclear, or acting upon information that is deemed useful.

Vignette 2

Michelle is a second-year internal medicine resident working in a large county hospital system. Confident in her own knowledge and skills, Michelle routinely takes charge of clinical planning and decision-making for patients on the ward team. She often has the correct management strategies on rounds, but she cannot articulate a broader and deeper clinical reasoning behind her decisions. In essence, she knows the "what" but not the "why." The ward attending expresses concern to the residency program director that although Michelle often knows the correct answer to some obscure recall questions, her deeper knowledge base and clinical skills are lacking. The attending believes Michelle's clinical reasoning and application of knowledge are behind expectations for her training level and documents this in the residency program's assessment system. In a meeting with the residency program director, Michelle discounts the assessment, stating "That attending just doesn't like me. I'm a strong resident with a good understanding of medicine." The program director discusses Michelle's performance on the most recent in-training exam, which was well below the 10th percentile nationally. Michelle notes that she was just really tired that day and reiterates that her knowledge base and clinical reasoning skills are excellent.

The program director wants to provide Michelle some coaching, especially around her biggest area of concern: Michelle's poor self-assessment skills that have led to overconfidence.

Thought Questions

1. When providing coaching, what data might be helpful for the program director to review with Michelle to help her recognize the overconfidence?

2. What communication strategies could the program director use to encourage deeper thinking and insight for Michelle?

3. How could the program director help Michelle learn about the differences between self-assessment and informed self-assessment?

Adjusting Phase

In the adjusting phase, learners must determine how to change their practice moving forward based upon their learning in the MAL process thus far. Adjusting practice includes consideration of how the individual will incorporate new learning into daily routines and practice when appropriate. At the core, the adjusting phase can be considered a change management problem. For small changes, there may be fewer logistic and emotional barriers involved in implementation (selecting a new antibiotic for a given infection based upon updated literature, for example). For larger changes, the individual must consider not just their own personal practice but also the system within which they provide care. Larger changes, such as how a physician might overhaul the care provided to an entire panel of diabetic patients, may require a more formal approach to change management like Kotter's model of change[2] from the business literature.

MASTER ADAPTIVE CONTINUOUS COGNITIVE SKILLS

To prepare to facilitate progress through the four phases of the MAL cycle, the learner must develop and then concomitantly leverage several core skills, all of which can be supported by coaches: critical thinking, reflection, self-monitoring, and metacognition.[3]

Critical Thinking

Critical thinking uses higher-order cognitive skills, such as conceptualization, analysis, and evaluation, and a deliberate disposition about thinking that leads to logical and appropriate action. Papp[4] and colleagues identify critical thinking as a "meta-competency that transcends other knowledge, skills, abilities, and behaviors required in health care professions," and have crafted developmental descriptors for the progression involved with acquiring critical thinking skills.

Reflection

Reflective skill can be defined as a "process that occurs before, during, and after situations with the purpose of developing greater understanding of both the self and the situation so that future encounters with the situation are informed from previous encounters."[5] This skill maximizes the learning benefit from various experiences and workplace encounters.

Self-Monitoring

Self-monitoring has been described as "the ability to notice our own actions, curiosity to examine the effects of those actions, and willingness to use those observations to improve behavior and thinking in the future."[6] Self-monitoring provides learners the skill needed to constantly assess the progress, or lack thereof, toward one's learning goals.

Metacognition

Metacognition is often referred to as "thinking about one's own thinking." It can be viewed as an overarching concept that synthesizes critical thinking, reflection, and self-monitoring. Metacognition allows individuals to focus not only on the outcome, but also "on the steps and decisions they make to achieve that outcome."[7]

Combining critical thinking, reflection, self-monitoring, and metacognition allows a learner to be intentional about their own learning and to understand whether their ongoing efforts are effective. Coaches should question and probe learner experiences in each of these essential cognitive skills and provide guidance and corrective direction as needed.

MASTER ADAPTIVE LEARNER BATTERIES

Several attributes are necessary to power the MAL cycle. The batteries[3] within the model describe four critical personal characteristics: curiosity, motivation, growth mindset, and resilience. Coaches can promote the learner's attention to each of these sources of learning power.

Curiosity

Curiosity represents the learner's internal desire to know and understand more. Curious learners are "less likely to accept what they are told uncritically, enjoy asking questions, and are more willing to reveal their questions and uncertainties in public."[8] They are driven to enter the learning cycle rather than leave questions unanswered.

Motivation

Self-determination theory differentiates between intrinsic and extrinsic motivation. High intrinsic motivation is "associated with better learning, better conceptual understanding, better academic performance and achievement, and higher levels of well-being than high extrinsic motivation."[9]

Mindset

An individual's belief about their own intelligence and capacity forms their mindset and directly affects their attitudes about learning, response to feedback, and response to setbacks. Dweck[10] differentiates individuals with fixed mindsets who believe that one's intelligence and talents are static and inherent from individuals with growth mindsets who believe abilities can be developed through one's dedication and hard work. Learners demonstrating a growth mindset invest in learning, accept critical feedback, and embrace challenges.

Resilience

Individuals often encounter difficulties or setbacks within the course of learning in both the classroom and clinical environments. Resilience is a complex construct that offers the ability to persist and continue in the learning process despite the encountered stress and challenges.[11]

Each of these personal characteristic batteries offer the opportunity for a coach to probe learner experiences in order to offer encouragement, reframe thinking, and develop targeted strategies.

MASTER ADAPTIVE LEARNER COACHING RHEOSTAT

Meaningful learning is hard.[12] The MAL process described previously can be labor intensive, especially for junior learners struggling to identify the most effective use of their time and energy. The expectation for development of adaptive expertise compounds this strain. Mylopolous and Regehr[13] describe a "clear burden" that adaptive expertise creates on learners by expecting them to stretch beyond routine expertise. Many learners have an inclination to master the basics first then consider evolving needs. Many raise questions ranging from "How can I actually learn in a way that develops adaptive expertise?" to "Is this effort worth it?" and even "Is it really my place to innovate (or prepare to innovate) in the health care setting?" But instilling MAL skills early, with the supportive scaffolding of a structured education program and external perspectives such as that of a coach, will position the learner for success over their entire career.

As noted in the lower portion of Fig. 2.1, the MAL model includes a coaching rheostat. Within the process, this is meant to indicate the valuable role of a coach in enhancing the efficiency and efficacy of the learning efforts. Although learning can (and does) happen without a coach, the process can be so much more impactful with effective coaching.

COACHING APPROACH FOR THE MASTER ADAPTIVE LEARNER PHASES

Coaching Skills in the Planning Phase

The coach's skill in prompting reflection by questioning the learner in targeted ways can be highly influential in the learner's selection of goals and learning strategies.

Vignette 3

Sandra is a busy junior faculty member working in an academic primary care clinic. Most of her administrative feedback to date centers around work productivity as measured by clinical revenue. During her yearly review with her division director, she comments that she finds it difficult to learn in the fast-paced environment and never really knows what to focus on during the few times she tries to set aside to "stay current with the literature." Her division director encourages her to meet with Eduardo, who serves as a coach for any interested divisional faculty.

In their first meeting, Sandra describes her frustrations with feeling stagnant in her professional development. She asks him if he could provide a list of readings that would help her improve her practice. Instead, Eduardo asks a series of questions, including "What was the last article you read?" "How did you select it?" and "How did your practice change?" Through his questioning, Eduardo recognizes that when Sandra spends time reading, it is typically haphazard and based on whatever article seems most interesting at the moment. Eduardo identifies a lack of planning for her learning, specifically the absence of any attempt to identify gaps in her own practice for focused learning and improvement. Eduardo suggests that planning and learning to address an identified gap in her practice would be more effective.

Thought Questions

1. What questions could Eduardo ask that would help Sandra focus on gaps within her own practice?
2. How could Eduardo incorporate data into helping Sandra identify gaps within her own practice?

There is evidence in medical education literature suggesting that, despite recognizing the importance of goal setting and planning, many learners struggle to manage their own learning process and desire guidance in this stage.[14]

Determining gaps and appropriate goals can be challenging for beginning learners. Although learning goals should be individualized and important to the learner, learners sometimes need guidance regarding what to focus on. Especially early on in training, knowing what you don't know is challenging. Learners often need to be encouraged to practice informed self-assessment, which includes looking at actual assessment data to trigger reflection, rather than relying solely on self-assessment, which has been repeatedly demonstrated as inaccurate.[15,16] Interpreting external performance evidence such as qualitative comments can be a challenge. The coach can facilitate meaningful use of data via probing questions such as "What do you think they meant by that comment?" or "How well did that evaluator know your work or abilities?" Guiding the learner to reflect on assessment evidence, articulate current educational opportunities, and incorporate their future career plans helps them identify priorities at any given point in time.

Once a gap is identified, learners can also benefit from coaching support in crafting the actual goal. Learners often start with a broad nonmeasurable goal; effective questioning by the coach can help hone in on the specific goal. Questions to ask include: "What will you be able to do when you achieve this goal?" "What do you mean by 'more comfortable/better at/more efficient/etc.?'" "How could you break that larger goal into smaller, more manageable goals?" Use of the ISMART mnemonic (Important, Specific, Measurable, Achievable, Relevant, and Time-Based) can help learners craft more effective learning goals. A scoring rubric[17] has been created to assess the quality of written learning goals. This rubric can be used as a feedback tool for learners to use on their own or as a prompt for discussion with the coach.

Another useful acronym for goal setting is WOOP,[18] which stands for Wish, Outcome, Obstacle, and Plan. This approach encourages learners to think not only about the goal they hope to accomplish (wish and outcome) but also to preemptively anticipate what will get in their way of meeting the goal and create a contingency plan to deal with barriers in the learning process. The benefit of WOOP is that it emphasizes the strategic planning skills needed in the planning phase in addition to goal setting. Studies[19-21] have found that creating and implementing a plan are the most difficult steps of goal setting for many learners. Strategic planning more than goal setting alone was most predictive of future outcomes. Coaches can play an important role in helping a learner consider barriers they might face with a particular goal and strategies to overcome them.

Another area ripe for coaching input in this phase is the selection of learning strategies to address a given goal. Often learners will resort to strategies they are comfortable with but that cognitive science shows do not result in deep long-term learning. By questioning the student about why they have chosen a given strategy, the coach can guide the student to select better learning strategies or even consider setting a goal around trying new strategies even though they are uncomfortable. Although coaches may suggest learning resources that they have found useful, learning preferences vary. Coaches don't need to be learning experts to support students in this arena, as even basic understanding of effective learning strategies and options available at their institution can be enough to facilitate this

conversation. Coaches can prompt the learner to think about whether their plan is realistic to carry out given the constraints of medical school.

Coaching Skills in the Learning Phase

The key role for a coach during the learning phase is to help assure the learner stays accountable to their goal. This can happen through regular conversations or brief check-ins via email or text. In addition, a coach can support a student in developing a broader network of people to support them in their learning. Students often worry that telling preceptors or teachers about their goals is a burden to teachers when, in fact, such direction can actually be a source of relief for teachers, assuring that their efforts are relevant to students' needs. Coaches can encourage students to view learning goals as a means of initiating conversation between students and teachers.

Coaching Skills in the Assessing Phase

The coach helps the learner make sense of feedback and assessment data to determine whether the learning plan has been effective. This involves reviewing the student's performance together and comparing it to the defined outcomes for the course or curriculum. The trusting relationship between the learner and coach is crucial for success in this process, as the learner must know that it is safe to talk about challenges and believes the coach approaches all conversations with the learner's best interest in mind. Much of this safety stems from separating coaching from grading.

Early in the relationship, the coach can ask the learner to reflect on what aspects of feedback and assessment seem accurate or perhaps "mostly" accurate. This acknowledges imperfections in performance evidence and can serve as a starting point to explore elements of agreement. Ideally, the learner identifies both critical and challenging feedback as well as the positives. If a learner is reticent to engage in the coaching relationship or lacks personal confidence, the coach can choose to focus initially on positive feedback and reserve the more critical feedback for a later time. Nevertheless, for the learner to grow, both the coach and learner must collectively address the critical feedback at some point.

A coach can help the learner see patterns in the feedback they have received and think critically about how best to actually change behavior in response to this feedback. Even if the quality of the feedback is poor (lacking specificity or clarity or is poorly worded/delivered), a skilled coach can help the learner reflect on what is written and think about ways to use the feedback to improve. In addition, the coach can help the learner figure out ways to seek out additional feedback on particular skills if the learner doesn't feel the feedback they have received is adequate or of sufficient quality.

Coaching Skills in the Adjusting Phase

The coach's key role in the adjusting phase is to promote reflection on the previous phases and help the learner determine how they want to move forward. A conversation about the adjusting phase can get into the nuances of what the student has learned and how they might approach future situations with slightly different contexts. Asking the student "what if" questions can help the student think about how best to implement the changes into their practice moving forward. Some desirable adjustments may involve interactions beyond the individual, in which case the coach can help the learner identify the leadership skills needed to enact broader change.

COACHING SKILLS RELATED TO THE BATTERIES THAT POWER THE MASTER ADAPTIVE LEARNER MODEL

Curiosity

The coach can help foster curiosity in the trainee by asking the trainee to describe what questions they still have after learning about a particular topic. In addition, the coach can model curiosity by asking the learner questions like "Why do you think that is?" or "Are there other ways of thinking about that?" The coach also needs to be aware that curiosity means some element of vulnerability and admitting what the learner knows and doesn't know. This can be challenging for some learners. Reaffirming that curiosity is beneficial supports deeper learning and learning that holds greater value to the trainee.

Motivation

Our educational system imposes many extrinsic drivers upon learners that can discourage engagement in the master adaptive learning process. Coaches can help learners recognize when they are excessively attentive to extrinsic motivations to the detriment of their long-term learning. One example would be a learner who invests too heavily in rote memorization as a strategy for enhancing performance on single best answer multiple-choice exams such as USMLE Step 1 or 2. While acknowledging the external driver, the coach can ask the trainee to reflect on whether that strategy was meaningful, sustainable, and fulfilling compared with the intrinsic motivation of learning needed to care for patients in the future. The coach could elevate the power of learning when one connects with patients: "How well do you remember material associated with the care of one of your patients?" "How often do you rely on rote

memorization in your work inside and outside of the medical arena?" Bonus coaching skill: How can the coach help the trainee see how curiosity and motivation are linked?

Mindset

Our educational systems create performance pressures that can perversely promote a fixed mindset, and coaches can help learners recapture a growth orientation. For a learner who is discouraged about ability, the coach can ask the trainee to reflect on times when the trainee was both a learner and a teacher. Can the trainee recall a time in the past when they struggled with, but eventually mastered, a difficult concept? How did that feel? Can the trainee, remembering a time they served as a teacher, give examples of how they leveraged multiple perspectives or approaches to help their learner grasp a challenging subject? Teaching a difficult concept to someone else demonstrates the growth mindset.

Resilience

At the level of professional training, many learners may have fused their academic success into their perception of self. A coach can help a trainee who has experienced a setback recognize the value of resilience by reflecting on examples outside of medicine. The coach can probe the trainee about past successes in different arenas—such as sports, music, or prior work experiences—that required resilience. Allowing the trainee to identify resilience in themselves and evaluate parallels to the current situation enables them to better envision and plan for success.

COMPETENCY-BASED MEDICAL EDUCATION

Competency-based medical education (CBME) provides a clarity of expectations and performance evidence that coaches can exploit to support learners at each stage of the MAL process. CBME is outcome driven, outlining the knowledge, skills, and attitudes necessary for successful practice to meet the needs of patients and communities. Those desired learning outcomes in turn direct the types of learning experiences necessary to support competency development and the types of assessments necessary to assure that competency is attained (Fig. 2.2). The core components of CBME[22] (Fig. 2.3) align well with the coach's role in assisting learners in engaging in the MAL model.

In CBME, the desired outcomes of the educational program are defined clearly. Competency milestones and entrustable professional activities (EPAs) are examples of methods currently in use to describe the desired outcomes of medical training, providing rich criterion-based behavioral descriptors of performance ranging from novice to expert. Given the breadth of competency demands

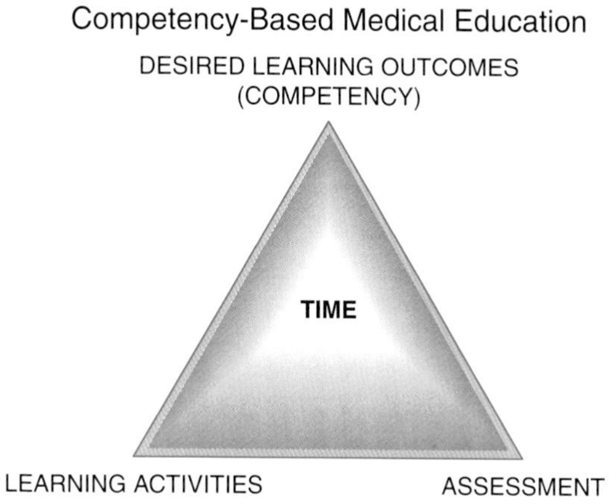

Competency-Based Medical Education

DESIRED LEARNING OUTCOMES
(COMPETENCY)

TIME

LEARNING ACTIVITIES   ASSESSMENT

Fig. 2.2 Competency-based medical education.

Core Components of Competency-Based Medical Eduction

Competency-Based
Medical Education (CBME)

Competency outcomes clearly
articulated (milestones, EPAs)

Developmental sequencing across
medical education continuum

Tailored learning experiences
in authentic roles

Competency-focused instruction based
on performance evidence

Programmatic assessment, with direct
observation and frequent feedback

Time as a resource

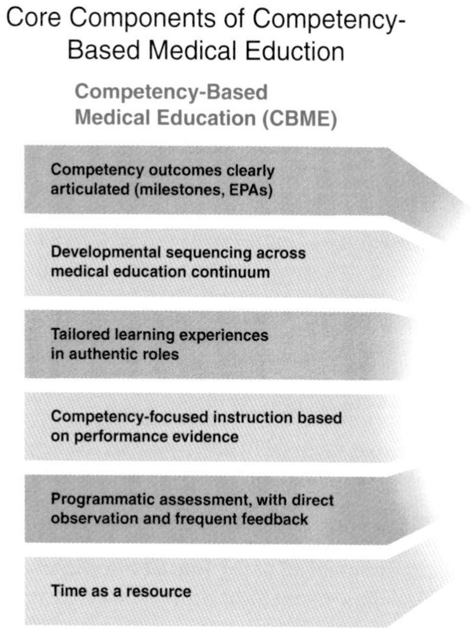

Fig. 2.3 Core components of competency-based medical education. *EPA*, entrustable professional activities. (Copyright American Medical Association.)

in health professions and the differing preparatory experiences and relative strengths of each student, the time and effort to develop any given competency will vary among students. Fidelity in implementation of CBME thus demands individualized pathways to enable each learner to optimize performance. Coaching is vital to support this

individualization and enable "precision education." The coach should encourage the learner to articulate goals in the context of the assessment system to which they are subjected. Alignment of personal goals with prevailing descriptions of performance expectations will facilitate the MAL assessing and adjusting phases.

In CBME, time becomes a resource for learning rather than a proxy measure of learning outcome. At every level of medical training, time is a precious and limited resource. Learners at any level of training can become overwhelmed by learning needs in a context of multiple competing demands on time and attention. Coaches serve an important role in helping learners focus their efforts. Established curricula in undergraduate medical education (UME) and graduate medical education (GME) are a starting point, offering developmental sequencing designed to support growth across the continuum. Many individual competency developmental needs can be met within the context of these existing learning opportunities, because most experiences offer a mixture of competency applications. For example, team-based classroom experiences aimed at fostering foundational knowledge also offer a chance to develop communication and teamwork skills. The coach can help the learner recognize the diverse learning opportunities embedded within standing coursework or rotations to identify paths to address their personal goals. In some instances, the coach may need to encourage a learner to advocate for tailored experiences in authentic roles to support their attainment of specific competency targets.

Successful CBME programs leverage programmatic assessment, an arrangement of assessment methods planned in a systematic way throughout a curriculum to support desired learning outcomes.[23] Ideally, the program provides frequent formative feedback and uses multiple objective measures of performance, including direct observation of authentic tasks that mimic the true work of the profession.[24] Coaches can draw upon this rich performance evidence arising from programmatic assessment to assist learners in a process of informed self-assessment. Helping the learner interpret feedback and identify performance trends that need attention is a vital role of the coach. Coaches should guide learners to seek appropriate competency-focused instruction based on performance evidence.

Because CBME expectations are criterion-based rather than normative, performance goals are framed relative to an ultimate performance level that can feel elusive to early learners. CBME frameworks do offer clarity regarding typical developmental pathways to competency. Examining competency milestones and descriptions of entrustable professional activities in detail illustrates a valuable perspective on growth that differs significantly from learners' common focus on immediate performance. The coach can prompt the learner to identify viable steps toward the ultimate performance level in order to track personal progress. Coaches can refer to these developmental trajectories to help learners recognize how new learning directly applies to practice and to encourage future competency aspirations. Early learners are likely to enact routine applications of new learning, but coaches can also help advanced learners recognize the need for novel applications and perhaps even the need to define new competencies required to meet evolving practice needs.

Coaches can leverage CBME frameworks to guide learners in each step of the MAL process—referring to clearly articulated competency expectations to direct the planning phase and to focus the learning phase for efficiency; leveraging rich performance evidence to guide the assessing phase; and highlighting a developmental framework to drive decisions of the adjusting phase. Coaches foster each learner's skills in self-regulation and self-directed learning that will be necessary to support continuous competency development throughout a career.

At the institutional level, coaching programs are resource intensive. Investments in coaching programs will be validated by alignment with the desired outcomes of the core educational program in addition to each learner's personal aspirations. Coaches should be informed regarding programmatic competency expectations in order to enhance the likelihood of achieving desired educational returns in the form of cohort competency development. Ideally, a coaching program includes regular opportunities for coaches to gather and share common challenges their learners face. This enables the team of coaches to elucidate programmatic gaps—areas in which entire cohorts of learners struggle to attain desired outcomes—and alert curricular leaders to the need for adjustment of learning opportunities. Such teams of coaches may also identify areas in which assessment data are limited or uninformative across an entire cohort of students and can advocate for revision of rubrics or assessment settings to improve the quality of the assessment system.

LEARNING ENVIRONMENT

The learning environment (LE) is a pervasive but often hidden influence on learning. We can define it as "the social interactions, organizational culture and structures, and physical and virtual spaces that surround and shape the learners' experiences, perceptions, and learning."[25] Because the LE is defined by the target and content of learning, it varies with the learning goals and the learners. It can be supportive of that learning or an obstacle to it—often concurrently.

In analyzing the influence of the LE, we find it helpful to think of it as having several dimensions and three hierarchical levels. The three dimensions are the physical, the virtual, and the social. The physical dimension encompasses buildings, rooms, heat, light, distracting noise, and soothing art objects. The virtual environment centers around the role of technology in education as it provides a virtual environment in a simulation center, online learning activities, spatially separated but interactive meetings, structured learning management systems, assessment dashboards, and digital learner portfolios. The electronic health record, so prominent a part of the clinical work environment, also becomes a major part of the clinical learning environment. Finally, the social dimension of the LE consists of three levels of organizational hierarchy: the individual and their character traits, experiences, abilities, and priorities, which make an experience of the LE different for everyone; the group and the interpersonal interactions that make it more or less functional for learning; and the organization with its policies, priorities, and incentives that influence education, even if intended for other purposes.

This conceptual framework helps us think about how the LE can support or hinder many of the points made earlier. For example, having asserted that the assessment program of a school is a source of useful feedback for identifying gaps and assessing learning outcomes, the coach must be mindful of the influence of the LE on assessment. If the LE around grading is highly competitive among students for honors recognition, it may direct attention away from using assessments for formative feedback and focus it instead on optimizing one's rank in the class. Improving such a competitive assessment environment to encourage a growth mindset might be done through a change to a pass-fail grading system.

Another LE factor could be the presence of student support services designed to assist learners dealing with the stresses of learning in medical school to avoid burnout. Environments without these institutional resources may be more at risk for adverse student outcomes and disruptive experiences that interfere with learning.

An effective coaching relationship with a learner must be built on trust. This trust is, in part, a relationship between the two individuals that will vary in strength depending on the "chemistry" between them. Thus the LE operates at a very small scale for individual coaching assignments. However, trust in the broader LE stems from an institutional transparency in processes and expectations and an improvement orientation of the educational

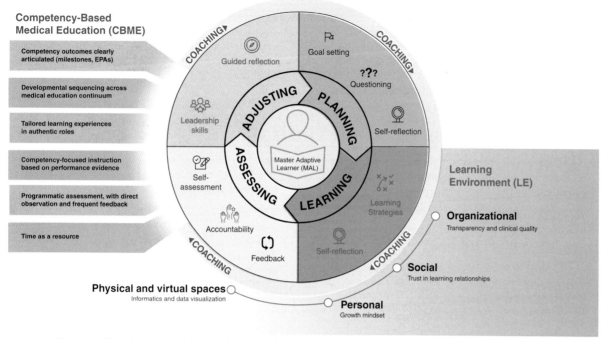

Fig. 2.4 Coaching, the Master Adaptive Learner model, and competency-based medical education are interwoven, and all rely heavily on a positive learning environment for success. *EPA,* entrustable professional activities. (Copyright American Medical Association.)

program itself. Educators must embrace student feedback just as students are asked to respond to faculty feedback. At the highest level, the LE may be systematically reduced or fostered depending on much larger dynamics, such as stability in leadership of the school or program, financial security of the institution, or active support for learners in need.

Student buy-in for master adaptive learning benefits from an LE in which faculty exhibit the self-examination and self-directed learning embodied in the MAL model. Coaches who understand the MAL model should strive to demonstrate how it works in the real world and how their own continuous learning is a key part of their professional identity. Conversely, faculty who are not self-aware or whose educational philosophy emphasizes the right answer rather than a good question will provide a chilling environment for the development of master adaptive learners. An LE can model curiosity and resilience through programming and communication strategies that highlight a diversity of expertise and acknowledge struggles as well as successes. Coaches can encourage students to identify connections throughout the environment that align with personal interests.

CONCLUSION

Coaching, the MAL model, and CBME are interwoven, and all rely heavily on a positive LE for success (Fig. 2.4). This relationship highlights potential messages conveyed by the LE. Coaching, like mentoring, is often a labor of love more than a path to riches. An organizational priority on compensating assessors and coaches for the time they devote to promoting learners' attainment of desired competencies and their development as master adaptive learners is a major environmental statement. Fostering the recruitment and retention of coaches requires training and ongoing support, which again comes from the organizational environment in the form of money, staff time, and other resources. Coaches can help students understand that the very existence of a supported coaching program is a sign of a positive learning environment designed to promote their individual success.

TAKE-HOME POINTS

1. The Master Adaptive Learner model offers a shared mental model for learners and coaches to facilitate meaningful growth and learning via the coaching process.
2. Precision education is enabled by the intersection of the Master Adaptive Learner model/competency-based medical education/coaching.
3. The learning environment and institutional culture are critical to support fidelity in the Master Adaptive Learner model/competency-based medical education/coaching.

QUESTIONS FOR FURTHER THOUGHT

1. How does the role of the coach need to change relative to the individual learner's skill in informed self-assessment and receptivity to the master adaptive learning process?
2. How can coaching serve as a scaffolding for competency development during formal training to instill self-directed habits throughout one's career?

ANNOTATED BIBLIOGRAPHY

Cutrer WB, Miller B, Pusic MV, et al. Fostering the development of master adaptive learners: a conceptual model to guide skill acquisition in medical education. *Acad Med.* 2017;92(1):70–75.
   This article presents the original description of the Master Adaptive Learner model.
Cutrer WB, Atkinson HG, Friedman E, et al. Exploring the characteristics and context that allow master adaptive learners to thrive. *Med Teach.* 2018;40(8):791–796.
   This article expands the context surrounding the Master Adaptive Learner model and how the different elements affect the learning.
Van Melle E, Frank JR, Holmboe ES, et al; International Competency-Based Medical Education Collaborators. A core components framework for evaluating implementation of competency-based medical education programs. *Acad Med.* 2019;94(7):1002–1009.
   This article clearly articulates the essential considerations for competency-based medical education programmatic implementation.
Gruppen LD, Irby DM, Durning SJ, Maggio LA. Conceptualizing learning environments in the health professions. *Acad Med.* 2019;94(7):969–974.
   This article presents a conceptual model for analyzing the learning environment and how it might interact with educational frameworks and activities, such as master adaptive learning.

REFERENCES

1. Cutrer WB, Miller B, Pusic MV, et al. Fostering the development of master adaptive learners: a conceptual model to guide skill acquisition in medical education. *Acad Med.* 2017;92(1):70–75.
2. Kotter JP. Leading change: Why transformation efforts fail? *Harvard Business Rev.* 1995:59–67 March/April.
3. Cutrer WB, Atkinson HG, Friedman E, et al. Exploring the characteristics and context that allow master adaptive learners to thrive. *Med Teach.* 2018;40(8):791–796.
4. Papp KK, Huang GC, Lauzon Clabo LM, et al. Milestones of critical thinking: a developmental model for medicine and nursing. *Acad Med.* 2014;89(5):715–720.
5. Sandars J. The use of reflection in medical education, AMEE Guide No. 44. *Med Teach.* 2009;31:685–695.
6. Epstein RM, Siegel DJ, Silberman J. Self-monitoring in clinical practice: a challenge for medical educators. *J Cont Educ Health Prof.* 2008;28(1):5–13.
7. Clark RC. Metacognition, self-regulation, and adaptive expertise *Building Expertise: Cognitive Methods for Training and Performance Improvement.* San Francisco, California: Wiley, Pfeiffer; 2008:313–321.
8. Deakin Crick R. Learning how to learn: The dynamic assessment of learning power. *Curric J.* 2007;18(2):135–153.
9. ten Cate O, Kusurkar R, Williams GC. How self-determination theory can assist our understanding of the teaching and learning processes in medical education. AMEE guide No. 59. *Med Teach.* 2011;33(12):961–973.
10. Dweck CS. *Mindset: the new psychology of success.* New York (NY): Random House Incorporated; 2006.
11. Dunn LB, Iglewicz A, Moutier C. A conceptual model of medical student well-being: promoting resilience and preventing burnout. *Acad Psychiatry.* 2008;32:44–53.
12. Brown PC, Roediger III, HL, McDaniel MA. *Make It Stick.* Cambridge, MA: Harvard University Press; 2014.
13. Mylopoulos M, Regehr G. How student models of expertise and innovation impact the development of adaptive expertise in medicine. *Med Educ.* 2009;43:127–132.
14. Nothnagle M, Anandarajah G, Goldman RE, Reis S. Struggling to be self-directed: residents' paradoxical beliefs about learning. *Acad Med.* 2011;86(12):1539–1544.
15. Sargeant J, Armson H, Chesluk B, et al. The processes and dimensions of informed self-assessment: a conceptual model. *Acad Med.* 2010;85(7):1212–1220.
16. Sargeant J, Eva KW, Armson H, et al. Features of assessment learners use to make informed self-assessments of clinical performance. *Med Educ.* 2011;45(6):636–647.
17. Lockspeiser TM, Schmitter PA, Lane JL, et al. Assessing residents' written learning goals and goal writing skill:

validity evidence for the learning goal scoring rubric. *Acad Med*. 2013;88(10):1558–1563.

18. Saddawi-Konefka D, Baker K, Guarino A, et al. Changing resident physician studying behaviors: A randomized, comparative effectiveness trial of goal setting versus use of WOOP. *J Grad Med Educ*. 2017;9(4):451.

19. Li ST, Paterniti DA, West DC. Successful self-directed lifelong learning in medicine: A conceptual model derived from qualitative analysis of a national survey of pediatric residents. *Acad Med*. 2010;85:1229–1236.

20. Li ST, Favreau MA, West DC. Pediatric resident and faculty attitudes toward self-assessment and self-directed learning: a cross-sectional study. *BMC Med Educ*. 2009;9:16.

21. Li ST, Tancredi DJ, Co JP, West DC. Factors associated with successful self-directed learning using individualized learning plans during pediatric residency. *Acad Pediatr*. 2010;10:124–130.

22. Van Melle E, Frank JR, Holmboe ES, Dagnone D, et al. International Competency-Based Medical Education Collaborators. A core components framework for evaluating implementation of competency-based medical education programs. *Acad Med*. 2019;94(7):1002–1009.

23. van der Vleuten CP, Schuwirth LWT, Driessen EW, et al. A model for programmatic assessment fit for purpose. *Med Teach*. 2012;34(3):205–214.

24. Carraccio C, Wolfsthal SD, Englander R, et al. Shifting paradigms: from Flexner to competencies. *Acad Med*. 2002;77(5):361–367.

25. Gruppen LD, Irby DM, Durning SJ, Maggio LA. Conceptualizing learning environments in the health professions. *Acad Med*. 2019;94(7):969–974.

3

Coaching Theories: A Scientific Foundation for Coaching Competencies in Medical Education

Margaret Moore

LEARNING OBJECTIVES

1. Explore coaching definitions.
2. Define how coaching competencies become science based.
3. Describe key coaching theories and tools.

CHAPTER OUTLINE

CHAPTER SUMMARY

Our goal for this chapter is to lay out a scientific foundation for coaching competencies in medical education, which are described in Chapter 4, and inspire interest in learning the coach approach. We start by reviewing coaching definitions described in the literature and then provide the definition of coaching in medical education that emerged from a 2018 coaching forum for medical educators. We then identify the main theories and tools that support the coaching competencies. This theoretical foundation for coaching in medical education provides a knowledge base for the next phase of this field—to fully educate medical educators in the knowledge and evidence base that supports basic coaching competencies and train and assess medical educators in basic coaching skills. This foundation supports the investigation of the impact of a standardized coaching approach on the well-being and professional development of medical students and residents. This chapter is also a call to continually evolve and refine both a scientific foundation and coaching competencies based on what is learned when studying coaching outcomes.

INTRODUCTION

Since 2000, a scientific foundation for the broad field of coaching has grown quickly, initially led by coaching psychology movements in Australia and the United Kingdom. Research in diverse areas that are addressed directly in coaching, including human motivation, self-efficacy, behavior change, psychological well-being, positive psychology, emotion regulation, and goal setting, has also flourished in the past two decades. Over the same timeframe, a significant body of literature has been published on the outcomes of coaching interventions in many domains, including leadership, the workplace, and health and well-being.

COACHING DEFINITIONS

History of Coaching Definitions

In the 1980s, coaching began its journey as a distinct discipline outside of sports. One of the pioneers, Sir John Whitmore, wrote the seminal 1992 book on coaching, *Coaching for Performance*,[1] drawing on Timothy Galwey's inner game model. Whitmore defined coaching: "Coaching is unlocking a person's potential to maximise their own performance. It is helping them to learn rather than teaching them—a facilitation approach." Whitmore asserted that coaching (in contrast to the knowledge download in teaching or training) is designed to help people cultivate self-awareness and personal responsibility.[2] Whitmore's video[3] demonstrating and comparing coaching and instruction in golf is legendary.

Vignette

Sue is a first-year medical student who reaches out to Evariste, a faculty coach, to get help with her test anxiety, which is interfering with her sleep and self-care. Her coach asks her to complete the science-based Values in Action character strength assessment, freely available at www.viacharacter.org, before their first coaching session, which is scheduled for an hour by way of video conferencing. Evariste starts by asking "What is going well for you, Sue?" This question helps Sue connect with her positive resources, which surprises her as she was ready to tell her coach about her anxiety in some detail to obtain problem-solving help. Sue reflects for a bit and mentions she has made a good friend, a classmate whom she feels close to, and they take power walks together on the weekend. Her coach reflects that he can feel her pleasure in this friendship and the outdoor exercise.

Then Evariste asks her to pause and take a couple of long, deep breaths. After a few moments he inquires, "If you were to imagine your best self, who would you be, what would that look like?" This is a new question for Sue; it draws out her autonomy and internal motivation. Sue responds by saying she would be calm and relaxed more of the time, enjoying learning and her classmates and not consumed with worry. Evariste continues to help Sue expand her envisioning and clarify her motivation on why being calm and relaxed is valuable and important to her.

Shifting the focus on helping Sue improve her confidence, Evariste asks, "What's an important challenge that you want to overcome that would help you become your best self?" Sue explains that she feels a great deal of family pressure to receive good grades. Her mother is a successful physician with high expectations. Sue is afraid of not meeting expectations, which makes her overanxious about tests and exams. Evariste empathically reflects his understanding of Sue's stressful situation. Then he asks about her top character strengths to help her with her recent challenges. "Love of learning" is her favorite, and together they brainstorm three possible new ways to apply her love of learning to overcome her anxiety, including trying out a new mindfulness technique, doing a short yoga routine when she doesn't have much time, and "changing the channel" to switch her thinking to learning something new rather than pleasing her parents. To turn the brainstorm into action, Evariste asks Sue to identify her action plan, which is to experiment with her three new habits in the next 2 weeks, with specific times and places scheduled. To close the session, he asks Sue to summarize and harvest what she has learned in that day's session. Sue notes that she was surprised by the power of imagining her best self and applying her love of learning in a creative way. She feels a lot better and expresses her gratitude for her coach's approach to empowering her to find her own way and step away from her parent's expectations.

Thought Questions

1. Which theories did the coach draw upon?
2. How does the coach support the learner's self-determination?
3. How does this conversation differ from counseling or mentoring?
4. How does this conversation compare with other approaches to supporting learners?

The first coaching psychologist, Anthony Grant, who founded the Coaching Psychology Unit at the University of Sydney in 2001, defined coaching psychology as "a branch of psychology that is concerned with the systematic application of the behavioral science of psychology to the enhancement of life experience, work performance and wellbeing for individuals, groups and organisations. Coaching psychology focuses on facilitating goal attainment, and on enhancing the personal and professional growth and development of clients in personal life and in work domains."[4]

In 2010, Moore and collaborators connected coaching to self-determination theory and positive psychology: "Coaching is a growth-promoting relationship which elicits internal motivation, leverages strengths, increases the capacity to change, and facilitates a change process through visioning, goal-setting, and accountability that leads to sustainable change for the good."[5]

Today, the International Coaching Federation, a global leader in accrediting coach training programs and credentialing coaches in life, business, and executive/leadership coaching defines coaching as "partnering with clients in a thought-provoking and creative process that inspires them to maximize their personal and professional potential."[6]

The formation in 2016 of the National Board for Health and Wellness Coaching (NBHWC),[7] a nonprofit affiliate of the National Board of Medical Examiners, led to the NBHWC definition of health and wellness coaching, which now supports American Medical Association Current Procedural Terminology (CPT) codes for health and well-being coaching services and the role of the coach as a nonphysician health care professional: "Health and wellness coaches work with individuals and groups in a client-centered process to facilitate and empower the client to develop and achieve self-determined goals related to health and wellness. Coaches support clients in mobilizing internal strengths and external resources, and in developing self-management strategies for making sustainable, healthy lifestyle, behavior changes."[8]

Over the past two decades, coaching definitions have been well-operationalized into coaching competencies, coach training, and education standards by credentialing organizations using best practices, including the International Coaching Federation, European Mentoring and Coaching Council, Association for Coaching, and the NBHWC.

Coaching Definition: Academic Coaching in Medical Education

Informed by a 2018 national thematic coaching meeting of invited medical educators and coaching experts and a review of the literature, this book's editorial team and others generated a definition of coaching, coaching theories (this chapter), and coaching competencies (Chapter 4).

The definition of coaching adapted for medical educators is "the art and science of facilitating sustainable change and growth of medical students and residents to realize their full potential as master adaptive learners. Key areas of change and growth include optimal learning, well-being, professional development and performance, and leadership."

Academic coaching is a process of facilitating self-awareness, discovery, and self-determination, in contrast to academic mentoring, which focuses on guiding and advising based on the mentor's expertise and experience. Coaches collaborate with coachees in a series of facilitative coaching sessions or meetings supporting the coachees, fully aligned with the Master Adaptive Learner model, to:

1. Articulate their personal visions (optimal future or ideal self), values (what is important and meaningful), strengths (what they do well that is a foundational resource), and goals (desired outcomes of the change process in terms of skills, behaviors, mindsets, and performance)
2. Expand curiosity and self-awareness, including evaluation of their strengths, skills, performance, and opportunities via review of objective assessments and feedback
3. Identify opportunities for change and development and strategies to address them
4. Design and evolve goals and an action plan
5. Be accountable to their commitments and reach their goals
6. Understand the benefits of coaching and self-coaching as resources for ongoing development throughout their careers

Academic coaching can also be delivered in "laser" coaching sessions, where coachees seek brief support, narrowing the focus of the previously mentioned steps to address a specific situation.

SCIENCE-BASED COACHING COMPETENCIES

Coaching draws on multiple and varied bodies of knowledge, as a synthesis of many theories, tools, and disciplines. Science-based coaching competencies integrate evidence-based theories and coaching tools that are relevant to the change or developmental process, including theories on self-determination, positive psychology (well-being and thriving), mindfulness, emotional intelligence, behavior change, goal setting, and navigating obstacles.

As a clear definition of a coaching domain matures, studies on coaching outcomes are completed and published, forming an evidence base for that coaching domain. For example, the most current review of executive coaching literature identified 15 randomized controlled studies and 11 categories of positive outcomes.[9] For health and wellness coaching, a 2018 compendium and a 2020 addendum of the literature[10,11] identified 108 randomized controlled studies and two meta-analyses in a wide variety of clinical populations, mostly showing clinically relevant outcomes (e.g., improvements in obesity, diabetes, hypertension, heart disease, chronic pain, cancer, and wellness).

Coaching for physician well-being includes three studies—one qualitative[12] and two randomized controlled studies (RCTs).[13] The two RCTs showed decreases in emotional exhaustion and other burnout symptoms, as well as improvements in quality of life, resilience, work engagement, psychological capital, and job satisfaction.

COACHING THEORIES

A core group of theories are widely applied in coaching, contribute a scientific base, and inform a toolbox for academic coaching competencies. The key theories and many of the tools supporting coaching have an extensive body of scientific literature behind them, including in some cases more than a thousand peer-reviewed studies. Many of these theories have validated assessments that can expand coachee self-awareness and insight and stimulate possibilities for growth. The abbreviated outlines in this chapter of the most widely used theories and tools are invitations to broaden and deepen learning.

Self-Determination Theory

At the core of the coaching approach is self-determination theory (SDT), a robust theory built over four decades by Edward Deci and Richard Ryan and now supported by numerous systematic reviews and meta-analyses.[14] SDT is focused on "fostering high quality motivation and performance, as well as psychological flourishing and growth."[15] SDT makes a scientific case for the facilitative approach of coaching (to empower rather than teach) and the purpose of coaching—empowering coachees to reach their highest level of motivation, engagement, creativity, persistence, competence, performance, and well-being.

Coaching is a well-being intervention in and of itself. Coaching directly serves the three primary psychological needs identified in SDT (autonomy, competence, relatedness), which are preconditions for well-being and autonomous self-regulation of behavior and growth. When these three needs are well-served, SDT studies find a full expression of human excellence and virtue. When these three needs are thwarted, psychological growth, functioning, and well-being are diminished and ill-being results. A good example of thwarted needs is burnout in the workplace resulting from inadequate relational support of autonomy and competence.

Core to SDT and coaching is autonomy support, empowering coachees to reflect upon and clarify their own coaching agenda, including visions, goals, and desired outcomes. Also core to SDT and coaching is serving the need for competence, facilitating growth in competence by helping coachees identify optimal challenges in which they value the potential outcome and have the capacity to effectively master the challenge with engagement.

In summary, the need to feel autonomous (rather than feel controlled), the need to feel competent (confident and effective), and the need to have supportive relationships (supporting autonomy and confidence though understanding the coachee's frame of reference in an open, trusting, authentic relationship) are directly served in coaching on the coachee's journey toward self-determination.

SDT also defines a range of motivation types, in particular distinguishing extrinsic motivation (e.g., awards, money, fame, status, social recognition), which has been shown to not improve well-being in lasting ways, from intrinsic motivation (e.g., acting in concert with one's values, serving others, personal growth), which leads to flourishing and more meaning in life. Intrinsic motivation is also one of the four batteries within the Master Adaptive Learner model that empowers the overall learning process, connecting SDT to the learner and their journey.

To note, the words "should," "ought to," or "must" are unintentional attempts to control motivation (by others or self) and do not support autonomy for the coachee in self-talk or coaching sessions.

What energizes and propels coachees forward is unimpeded access to their intrinsic motivation. Ryan and Deci summarize: "Intrinsic motivation is the spontaneous propensity of people to take interest in their inner and outer worlds in an attempt to engage, interact, master, and understand, without needing external rewards."[14] The role of coaches is then to help coachees tap into and harness their intrinsic motivation to grow their competence, performance, and well-being. The coachee's level of motivation and self-efficacy are key predictors of goal initiation and sustainability over time.

Unconditional Regard

Unconditional regard in coaching means that coaches accept and value coachees without conditions or contingents, which supports and satisfies coachees' autonomy needs. Ryan and Deci note, "Coaches who can be curious and engaged in the coachee's thoughts, perceptions, and experiences are likely to be met with more trust, more energy, and more satisfaction in the relationship."[15]

Unconditional regard is also a precondition for psychological safety, when the coachee feels safe to authentically share their values, experiences, perspectives, and concerns with the coach, and feels safe to explore difficult topics such as feedback, conflicts, or equity and inclusion issues.

To give unconditional regard, coaches learn to set aside their controlling natures—ego involvements, biases, judgments, and agendas concerning the direction and outcomes of coaching. Coaching gives space to the coachee's full autonomy in making reflective and well-informed choices about their direction and challenges.

Curiosity

Curiosity—the desire to know and understand—is a powerful intrinsic motivator for learning, behavior, creativity, and growth.[16] It is another one of the four batteries of the Master Adaptive Learner model. Open-minded curiosity about self, others, and the world can be generated for its own intrinsic sake, and it can be fueled by an autonomous interest in resolving challenges.[15]

Important to coaching, when a coachee's needs for autonomy are met, curiosity increases.[17] Coaches can further expand a coachee's curiosity through genuine and varied open questions, posed in a mindful tone that clearly communicates no agenda, preference, bias, expectation, judgment, or any other unintentional controlling behavior.

Motivational Interviewing

Motivational interviewing (MI), which is widely taught to clinicians to help them shift from an expert advisory role to a facilitative role, can be described as "SDT in conversation." MI is an evidence-based theory centered on conversational techniques[18] that engage a coachee's sense of autonomy, curiosity, motivation, competence, and creativity and can include:

- Open inquiry (asking open, curious, provocative questions to generate awareness and insight)
- Active listening (listening with undivided attention and interest for the other's words, thoughts, emotions, perspectives, frame of reference, and meaning)
- Reflections (to confirm listening and expand the coachee's reflection)
- Affirmations (to affirm strengths, virtues, values, and progress)
- Summaries (to bring clarity to complex issues)

As in SDT, a key principle of MI is to evoke intrinsic motivation for change, rather than extrinsic motivation (e.g., from a coach, boss, or family member), which can inadvertently trigger resistance to change when another's agenda is imposed. MI includes a technique called "rolling with resistance" when a coach has inadvertently "stepped on" the coachee's autonomy. To respond to the coachee's

resistance, the coach adopts the coachee's frame of reference, with unconditional regard, showing acceptance and acknowledging that the coachee's perspective is valid.

Another MI tool is called a "ruler," a 1 to 10 qualitative self-assessment on a coaching question that generates self-awareness; for example, how motivated or confident are you on these actions for next week on a scale of 1 to 10 (self-insight)? Why is the score not lower (pulling out strengths and confidence)? What would be an optimal score (ideal self)? What would it take to increase your score by one point (optimal challenge)? A general rule is for coachees to have a score at 7 or above for both motivation and confidence before proceeding into action.

In summary, MI facilitative techniques draw out the coachee's reflections, ideas, and insights rather than close them off with judgment, instruction, and advice, thereby serving the coachee's autonomy and competence. Coachees can then reflect and clarify their focus for change and their intrinsic reasons for change, and commit to their desired changes.

Intentional Change Theory

Intentional change theory (ICT) is a leadership coaching model developed by Richard Boyatzis and collaborators as a direct application of SDT.[19] ICT has five steps for self-change:

1. Discover one's vision for one's ideal self
2. Understand the gap between the real self today and the desired future self
3. Create a learning agenda to move toward one's ideal self
4. Experiment with and practice new habits
5. Get support from the coach as well as other social and environmental resources.

In concert with step 2, the Master Adaptive Learner model includes "gap" identification in the planning phase.

In a *Leadership Quarterly* article, the authors identify ICT principles that apply SDT and summarize: "Leadership coach facilitated discovery of future ideal self, present real self, learning agenda, and experimentation, meet a leader's needs for autonomy, relatedness, and competence."[20]

A coaching process that is similar to ICT—also aligned with SDT in fully exploring the coachee's vision, values, strengths, challenges, creativity, and action steps—is foundational for science-based health and wellness coaching.[21]

Advice and Feedback in Coaching

In coaching, giving feedback and advice is secondary to the facilitative process in which the coach supports the coachee's self-discovery around their autonomy, values, motivation, desired outcomes and goals, strengths, and challenges that they are interested in overcoming. In certain situations, there is value in the coach offering information, advice, or feedback to a coachee. For example, some of the science around behavior change, thriving, and growth may be valuable and may not be known by a coachee. A brief just-in-time description of a topic (e.g., coaching tool rationale, autonomous motivation, positive emotions, or growth mindset) can be valuable and timely information for the coachee to consider. The coach's authentic observations of the coachee's experience are important to coachee learning. The coachee may receive feedback from others that is important to their professional development, and that can be safely and productively explored in a coaching session.

The coach's purpose in sharing information, advice, or feedback is to inform the coachee in order to support self-awareness and competence development and expand the range of possibilities. It is important for the coach to ask permission to offer information—"would you be interested in…"—preserving a coachee's autonomy in making choices. Then the coach may convey the information openly and empathically as information to consider, not as a request, judgment, or criticism.[15]

Positive Psychology

Positive psychology was founded in 1998 in part to provide a scientific counterbalance to all that goes wrong with mental health, for example, as laid out in the *Diagnostic and Statistical Manual of Mental Disorders,* fifth edition. The field emerged as "the scientific study of the strengths that enable individuals and communities to thrive. The field is founded on the belief that people want to lead meaningful and fulfilling lives, to cultivate what is best within themselves, and to enhance their experiences of love, work, and play."[22] Positive psychology has strongly influenced coaching since its beginning, including the launch of a coaching specialty called positive psychology coaching.

Character Strengths

An early seminal positive psychology book, *Character Strengths and Virtues: A Handbook and Classification,* describes the 24 "character strengths and virtues" explored in a 5-year scholarly endeavor to investigate the science, philosophy, and religious origins of these strengths.[23] This book is a key reference in coaching and foundational to the Master Adaptive Learner model (Chapter 2), which specifically includes curiosity, perseverance (resilience), and self-regulation (self-monitoring), and more generally includes creativity, open-mindedness, love of learning, judgment, and humility.

The scientific investigation of character strengths has been widely expanded and disseminated globally. The evidence-based Values in Action Character Strengths assessment (www.viacharacter.org) provides a starting point for coachees who are new to self-assessments and want to understand and apply their most important values to their change efforts (Fig. 3.1). It also supports coaching conversations on using one or more character strengths in new ways to address challenges or improve performance and well-being.

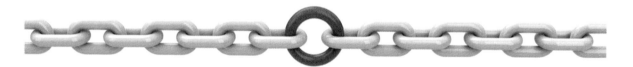

wisdom & knowledge	Creativity, Curiosity, Open-mindedness, Love of learning, Judgment
courage	Honesty, Bravery, Perseverance, Zest
humanity	Kindness, Love, Social Intelligence
justice	Fairness, Leadership, Teamwork
temperance	Forgiveness, Humility, Prudence, Self-regulation
transcendence	Appreciation of beauty, Gratitude, Hope, Humor, Spirituality

CHARACTER
VALUES in ACTION
www.viacharacter.org

Fig. 3.1 Classification of Character Virtues and Strengths. (Copyright 2004–2021, VIA Institute on Character. www.viacharacter.org.)

Positive Emotions

Three decades of research on positive emotions by Barbara Fredrickson, who founded the University of North Carolina Positive Emotions and Psychophysiology Laboratory, have demonstrated the positive psychological, cognitive, and physiologic impact of cultivating positive emotions and sharing them socially as a daily activity.[24] Applying Fredrickson's "broaden and build theory," when a coach invites a coachee to identify and amplify positive experiences and emotions, the coachee is more open-minded and creative and more willing to take risks. Over time, continued cultivation of positive emotions builds resources, including physical health, resilience, and better relationships, which further supports coaching as an intervention for well-being.

Positive emotions are then vital resources for navigating self-change and improving well-being. Coaching conversations can incorporate positivity assessments (e.g., positivityratio.com) and intentionally elicit and harvest positive emotions—for example, asking what is going well, what is the best thing that happened, what you are learning, what would inspire you, etc.

Psychological Capital

Since the early 2000s, the term *psychological capital* has emerged to describe evidence-based resources that support resilience, positive change, well-being, and positive organizational cultures. The acronym HERO—hope, efficacy, resilience, and optimism—represents psychological capital, describing the resources that, to date, have a scientific foundation.[25] The benefits of fostering psychological capital in academic settings have been explored.[26] PsyCap, as it is called, is a mediator in reducing student stress and improving well-being, along with two other mediators, self-compassion and social support.

Appreciative Inquiry

Appreciative inquiry (AI) is a strengths-based process developed by psychologist David Cooperrider when he was studying the "appreciative" culture at the Cleveland Clinic for his PhD program. The AI process has five steps[27] and has been introduced to medical education[28] and is widely used in coaching. A coach guides the coachee through an inquiry that intentionally "appreciates the good" in order to amplify resources that support positive change. The first step is to unpack positive past experiences in a particular area of interest (e.g., academic learning or clinical empathy), followed by identifying the strengths engaged and the generative conditions that enabled the best experiences. Then the coachee defines a vision or dream of being at one's best, followed by an action plan to apply the strengths and conditions to move toward the vision.

Essentially, AI helps the coachee understand what empowers them to be at their best and learn how to make their best experiences more frequent and consistent. As Cooperrider notes: "What you appreciate, appreciates."[29] It's worth noting that the AI process doesn't have a step for addressing challenges; AI focuses on building on the good—existing strengths and best experiences—in contrast to other tools where a vision is developed that surpasses lived experiences to date or where obstacles are explicitly navigated as growth opportunities.

Growth Mindset

Carol Dweck's work on the growth mindset aligns with positive psychology as it improves human thriving and accomplishment. "When people exhibit a growth mindset, a belief that they have the potential to get better with hard work, good strategies and help from others, set more challenging goals in life and pursue those goals longer. When people operate from a fixed mindset, believing they cannot change their talents and strengths, they believe that they have limited potential to improve and set less challenging goals."[30]

People generally experience a mix of both fixed and growth mindsets in their lives, and coaches help coachees continually cultivate a growth mindset, viewing challenges, obstacles, and barriers to change as opportunities to learn, grow, and accomplish more. This isn't a new perspective; the Greek Stoics advised: "the obstacle is the way." Leaning into challenges is a productive path to growth for coachees when they operate from a growth mindset and have a coach's support of autonomy and competence.

Mindfulness

Given the core function of expanding self-awareness, mindfulness—which integrates metacognition, observing, and exploring one's own thinking and feeling—is an important domain to coaching as well as to being a master adaptive learner (Chapter 2). Mindfulness is defined by Jon Kabat-Zinn: "Mindfulness is awareness that arises through paying attention, on purpose, in the present moment, nonjudgmentally, in the service of self-understanding and wisdom."[31]

Deci and Ryan summarize the self-determination perspective on mindfulness: "The power of mindfulness to clarify goals and support autonomous regulation has been confirmed in numerous studies. People higher in mindfulness had better access to their emotional states, were more vital and autonomously motivated, and showed greater congruence between implicit and explicit emotions. People with more mindful awareness responded less defensively to threats, suggesting that more mindful awareness can be considered an important underpinning for mental health and well-being."[15]

In close alignment with the Master Adaptive Learner model, coaching sessions can be reasonably described as mindfulness in action, helping coachees observe themselves and the world, expand their awareness and self-understanding (noticing their inner dynamics and values), and access meta-awareness and insight or wisdom (stepping back or detaching from their inner dynamics to witness themselves and others more objectively).

Among the wide variety of mindfulness interventions and applications described in the literature is a 2019 systematic review of the impact of mindfulness-based interventions on doctors' well-being and performance,[32] mostly showing positive effects on performance and well-being (enhanced understanding of self and others).

The five-factor mindfulness assessment[33] can be readily translated into coaching questions:

1. Awareness (not automatic pilot, not suppressing or minimizing)
   What are you noticing about your present state—your thoughts, emotions, actions, physical sensations?
2. Observing (no interpretation, no exaggerating)
   What are you observing (without evaluation) about how you feel or what you are thinking?
3. Describing (labeling with granularity)
   What words would you use to describe the emotions (or thoughts) that you are experiencing?
4. Nonjudgment (acceptance)
   What does/would it feel like to accept (not judge) the contents of your awareness—your thoughts, emotions, sensations, and actions?
5. Nonreactivity (not carried away)
   What would it look like to pause and not react to the contents of your mind in this moment, to simply observe?

A mindfulness framework particularly relevant to coaching is called S-ART, which stands for self-awareness, self-regulation, and self-transcendence.[34] It maps well to the change process, starting with self-awareness, followed by self-regulation, leading to self-transcendence, when one has outgrown old patterns of emotions, thoughts, and behaviors.

Self-insight, defined as the clarity of one's understanding of one's thoughts, feelings, and behavior, is a metacognitive factor central to the process of purposeful, directed change and meaning making. Self-insight as depicted as one's "ideal self" is a particularly valuable self-insight in coaching.[35]

When a coach brings a mindful presence (aware, open, curious, observing, accepting, compassionate), coachees become more mindful—more aware, open, and accepting of their values, opportunities, and challenges and more able to pause, self-regulate, and make new choices, which is important in the change process.

EMOTIONAL INTELLIGENCE

Theory of Constructed Emotions

Many scientists have endeavored to help us better understand and navigate emotional states. A new theory of constructed emotions[36] teaches that the brain automatically constructs emotions, based on past experiences, to communicate the brain's evaluations and predictions of the balance of demands and resources moment to moment. Emotions are not produced in direct response to the internal or external environment, and they are not reflections of objective reality. Emotions are signals from the brain to act, to meet internal needs, or to seek learning. Hence there is much value to mindful self-observation by coachees in understanding, navigating, and learning from their emotional states.

Emotional Intelligence

Emotional intelligence (EI) emerged in the mid-1990s and is defined as the ability to understand and regulate one's own emotions, understand others' emotions, react to both in a productive way, use these skills to make good judgments, and avoid or solve problems. There are numerous EI assessments used in coaching, including the Emotional Quotient Inventory (EQI), which has been studied in graduate medical education.[37] A core coaching competency is helping coachees navigate their emotions and the emotions of others in their relationships and teams, applying mindfulness-based inquiry.

Self-Compassion

Adding to the five mindfulness factors, the emerging field of self-compassion is important in coaching and being widely applied in mindfulness practices. Its founder, Kristin Neff notes: "Self-compassion entails being gentle, kind, warm, and understanding toward ourselves when we suffer, fail, or feel inadequate, rather than ignoring our pain or flagellating ourselves with self-criticism."[38] Coaches help coachees develop not just self-acceptance, but also self-compassion toward their emotional states and circumstances, which improves self-regulation and equanimity and increases compassion toward others.

Acceptance and Commitment Coaching

Acceptance and commitment therapy[39] (ACT) is applied by coaches in leadership and well-being and is also described as emotional agility.[40] ACT extends mindfulness (noticing, stepping back to observe oneself with acceptance) and self-compassion (being kind and gentle to oneself) to add two more steps. One step is identifying one's core values (what matters right now? who do I want to be?). Emotions can be signposts of values that are not being served. The second step is committing to take action aligned with one's values. All together these steps create psychological flexibility—the ability to be fully conscious, embrace our emotional experiences, and be guided in our actions by our heartfelt values. Psychological flexibility contrasts with being hooked and controlled by emotions or being rigid or ruminating, which can lead to a downward spiral of burnout, depression, and other clinical symptoms.

Nonviolent Communication

Nonviolent communication[41] is a widely used tool in coaching and has four steps for efficiently processing and learning from emotions. The coachee first shares a troubling story, laced with both factual and emotional content. Then the coach asks the coachee to separate the facts from the arising emotions, retelling the story as a factual narrative without emotions. The coachee then identifies and names the emotions that initially accompanied the facts. Then the coachee identifies the unmet needs conveyed by each emotion and makes requests to themselves or others to meet the unmet needs.

To summarize, some coaching questions that foster EI include:
1. What does it feel like to appreciate and open up fully to your emotional experiences?
2. What are your best experiences of self-compassion? What enables you to feel self-compassion? How could you activate those enablers now? (This is also an example of the step in AI of unpacking the generative conditions of best experiences.)
3. What values do you hold that are important in this moment? If you were to take action aligned with those values, what would that look like?
4. What supports you in being compassionate toward others? When are you at your most compassionate? When are you at your least compassionate?
5. What messages do you think this emotional state is sending to you?

TRANSTHEORETICAL MODEL OF CHANGE

When coachees decide on their agenda for positive change, the coach has an opportunity to help them better understand and improve their readiness to change. The Transtheoretical Model of Change (TTM) has mapped the readiness to change a behavior into five stages of change that are important as coaches help coachees identify their goals:
1. Precontemplation—no way!!! Very low confidence or defiance
2. Contemplation—on the fence. Maybe . . . Maybe not
3. Preparation—getting ready, planning, anticipating

4. Action—actively engaging effortfully in new behaviors and mindsets while still vulnerable to lapses
5. Maintenance—behaviors and mindsets become easier and mostly automatic

Readiness to change a behavior is a predictor of change success (the higher the readiness the more likely success). Readiness is determined by a decisional balance—the balance of the pros for change (motivation) and the cons or barriers to change (which reduce confidence), aligned well with SDT's core needs of autonomy and confidence.

A meta-analysis showed that the two drivers of the change process are consistent across 48 health behaviors and reasonably extrapolated to other behaviors.[42] Figure 3.2 shows that the combination of the level of motivation and barriers (driving confidence) determine readiness to change on any given behavior and are behavior specific. Further, basic research has generated a rule of thumb in behavior change,[43] which is that most people are not ready to change most behaviors: approximately 40% of people are in precontemplation, 40% in contemplation, and 20% in preparation. The TTM lesson for coaching is that most coachees benefit from broader inquiry and deeper reflection on their motivation (intrinsic reasons to change) and confidence (identifying and overcoming obstacles) in order to be successful in behavior change.

In this regard, SDT and the transtheoretical model point coaches toward awareness-generating conversations on the decisional balance of motivation and confidence or competence. This can be a simple analysis where the coachee first lists all of the reasons to change (motivation) and then all of the reasons not to change (obstacles that reduce confidence). Another approach is to alternate back and forth between one reason to change and one reason not to change, an application of the Wish, Outcome, Obstacle, Plan (WOOP) tool described later. Both techniques quickly

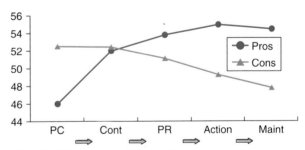

Fig. 3.2 The pros and cons of changing across stages of change for 48 behaviors. Precontemplation (PC), Contemplation (Cont), Preparation (PR), Action, and Maintenance (Maint). (From Hall KL, Rossi JS. Meta-analytic examination of the strong and weak principles across 48 health behaviors. *Prev Med.* 2008;46(3): 266–74.)

help coachees amplify motivation and understand what obstacles to focus on, which generates direction for strategizing on what will overcome key obstacles and build confidence. In alignment, the Master Adaptive Learner model has an "adjusting phase" that teaches change management strategies to address challenges in the change process.

GOAL SETTING

SDT posits that goal setting be informed by the notion of optimal challenges. Goals that are not too easy (which could dissipate interest), and at the same time not so stressful or demanding as to impair confidence, provide an optimal challenge. Optimal goals and plans that can be mastered with motivated persistence are also best chosen by the coachee, in full expression of their autonomy. Self-monitoring of goal progress also helps a coachee become more autonomous and competent.[15]

A scientific review of goal setting in coaching[44] presents highlights of how best to approach behavior change with coachees:

SMART Goals

Behavioral goals that are specific, measurable, achievable, relevant, and time based are broadly recommended in behavior change efforts, as they have been shown to be more concrete and effective (I will do 5 minutes of deep breathing at 8 a.m. and 8 p.m. on Mondays, Wednesdays, and Fridays) than broad goals statements (such as, I want to manage stress better).

Challenging Goals

In contrast, countering the approach of setting realistic behavioral goals is research that suggests that more challenging goals are more motivating and stimulating initially, leading to greater effort, focus, and persistence than moderately difficult goals. Later though when challenges emerge, reducing the goal challenge may be important for success.

Optimal Challenge

For some coachees, ambitious goals may be more motivating; for others, ambitious goals can seem too hard and deplete confidence. The optimal level of goal challenge can also vary for an individual coachee, as motivation and competence vary across one's professional and life domains.

Short-Term Goals

Better outcomes are accomplished with short-term goals than long-term goals, as they increase motivation and self-regulation more than long-term goals and are optimally chunked into smaller steps.

Progress Tracking

Writing out short-term goals, as well as progress tracking and communicating progress to others, including a coach, increases behavior change success.

Deliberate Practice

Plenty of deliberate practice, supported by a clear action plan (defining what, when, where, how) contributes to success, unless the coachee doesn't have sufficient capabilities for target behaviors and success may be unrealistic. It may then be better to support coachees in shifting to more attainable goals.

Backup Plans May or May Not Be Helpful

Having backup plans may be helpful, but some studies show that they can dampen motivation.

Social Support and Emotion Regulation

Some research indicates that the availability and type of social support and emotion regulation are equal or more important to behavior change than thinking about goals.

Negative Feedback Can Reduce Motivation

Negative feedback from others can elicit stress and increase cortisol levels, which reduce motivation and readiness to change; hence it's vital to provide feedback to coachees with permission and in the positive context of an opportunity to move toward their autonomous vision and desire for growth and use their strengths in new ways.

In summary, it is important for coaches to help coachees define their optimal scale and timeframe of their visions and goals and translate goals into their choice of behaviors and action.

WOOP

Gabriele Oettingen developed the four-step WOOP behavior change tool, starting first with the coachee identifying their vision or wish.[45] The second step is having the coachee define the desired outcome. The third step is to define the main obstacles. The fourth step is to develop a plan to overcome obstacles, and the goals emerge as ways to implement these strategies. This tool ensures that goals aren't clarified until the first three steps are complete and that goals are focused on overcoming obstacles and increasing confidence. WOOP has been shown to deliver better outcomes than simple goal-setting for physician residents.[46]

GROW

The GROW tool popularized by Sir John Whitmore is a four-step inquiry.[1] First, the coachee decides where they wish to go (the goal) and describes where they are currently (reality). Then the coachee explores various routes (the options) to the goal destination. In the final step, the coachee commits to the plan of action and prepares for obstacles on the way (the way forward).

NAVIGATING CHALLENGES

All of the theories and tools introduced so far provide a basic scientific foundation for facilitating conversations to help coachees:

1. Clarify the direction of change—a desired wish, dream, or vision of optimal/future self, aligned with their intrinsic motivation, including personal values and purpose
2. Clarify the challenges to be navigated and behavioral goals or action plans to move forward that address challenges by experimenting with and practicing new habits
3. Cultivate the resources needed to support the change process—including mindfulness for self-awareness and self-regulation, effective harvesting of emotional experiences, a growth mindset, psychological capital (hope, optimism, resilience, efficacy), and amplifying positive emotions and strengths

Last but not least, there are approaches designed to help coachees bring a deep, curious focus during a coaching session to navigating a growth opportunity or challenge (a growth edge) to enable self-discovery and expand possibilities. Once basic coaching skills are mastered, the gift to coaches is to facilitate generative conversations, using simple or more advanced tools, that lead to perceptible shifts in awareness, learning, perspectives, and competence. These are the peak moments of coaching, enhancing the mastery and well-being of coaches.

Generative Moments

Coaches encourage coachees to identify an agenda for a coaching session, a growth opportunity that they are ready to explore. This opens the door to a "generative moment," an energetic, creative conversation, described as relational flow or the intuitive dance, where the coach helps coachees explore new ideas and vantage points freely until they experience a small shift in learning, insight, perspective, or attitude that perceptibly increases their confidence in overcoming a challenge.[21] The accumulation of small shifts over weeks, months, and beyond can lead to "quantum shifts,"[47] which are shifts in identity—for example, "I am not the kind of person who goes to bed early to make time for wellness activities early in the morning" to "I can't wait to go to bed early so that I can start the new day calm and energized after a fast walk."

To navigate generative moments, coaches select open-ended coaching questions, such as "What would be the outcome if you overcame this challenge?" Coaches also adapt quickly when questions don't lead anywhere; they flexibly change to a different tool. Possible tools explored in this chapter include AI, decisional balance or mental contrasting, nonviolent communication, and applying character strengths in novel ways. To add, simple brainstorming can work well where the coachee and coach each take turns offering ideas, the more unconventional at first the better. A creative way to elicit nonlinear thinking is for the coach to ask the coachee to make a quick association between their challenge and a surprising, random object (like a table or a tiger). The coachee then shares new ideas that come up. The generative discussion has served its purpose in a coaching session when the coachee's motivation and confidence are boosted.

Hope psychology suggests that hope (and confidence) increases when people have generated at least three new ideas or strategies to address a challenge, giving them more hope so that they have the creative ability to identify more strategies if the first three don't succeed.[48]

Cognitive Behavioral Coaching

Cognitive behavioral coaching[49] starts with guided discovery, sometimes called Socratic questioning,[50] that increases the coachee's self-awareness of how their thinking, emotions, and behaviors are operating and getting in the way of the change progress. The coachee begins to understand how their beliefs and perspectives determine and distort their mindsets and reactions. The coach helps the coachee reframe and consider new perspectives and then experiment with new mindsets and behaviors. For example, the veracity of "I feel like an imposter" is tested and then recognized as unproductive. The coachee decides to reframe the perspective as "I'm grateful for this intensive learning phase," which the coachee brings to mind when the imposter thought arises. Eventually the grateful frame becomes the dominant response.

Immunity to Change

The immunity to change tool is an advanced form of cognitive behavioral coaching. It is based on the subject-object theory in adult development, which in brief is the simple mechanism by which adults develop maturity through processing life experiences, moving elements in their minds from subject to object.

When your mind is "subject" to an assumption, belief, perspective, or emotional state, it is in effect controlled, as if your mind is a puppet and the puppeteer is the subconscious subject. You are not aware or awake to this implicit control. You take it as reality. Like in the S-ART model discussed in the mindfulness section, at some point, you become aware that the assumption or belief may not be functional or true, and you begin to observe it by accessing meta-awareness. In this step, the subject becomes object; it is now an object of your attention, something that can be seen, even if it still controls you. With time and exercises (like the immunity to change model about to be described), the object can be integrated, where your mind is no longer controlled by the original "subject" and your consciousness has expanded.[51]

The immunity to change tool developed by Robert Kegan and Lisa Lahey is a set of four practical steps that allows you to move one or more subjects controlling your mind and behavior (holding back your desire to improve) to objects, and then you can transcend and outgrow the original assumptions and beliefs.[52] It is particularly important when other change tools have not been effective and can be helpful in the Master Adaptive Learner model "adjusting phase." The four steps for a coachee are:

- Select a desired area for improvement where motivation is high (e.g., getting better at listening to improve relationships) and improvement has been elusive for a while.
- Identify one or several countering or sabotaging behaviors that get in the way of the desired improvement (e.g., distracted by own problems, thinking about how best to respond, aroused emotions).
- Explore the underlying assumptions and worries (the bad things that will happen if I don't do the sabotaging behavior) that drive the countering behaviors (e.g., if I don't prepare to respond I won't have anything useful to say, my problems are more pressing than this conversation). These assumptions drive the behaviors that create an immunity to change.
- Develop experiments to test the assumptions behind the sabotaging behaviors (e.g., test setting one's problems aside when listening for 2 minutes at a time to

check whether anything bad happens). Over time a set of tests can overturn the implicit assumptions and the immunity to change.

COACH DEVELOPMENT

Shift from Expert to Coach

Our last section in this chapter moves the spotlight to the coach's development, which is a lifelong journey of growth in maturity and impact. The switch in roles from teacher, mentor, or adviser to facilitative coach is a 180-degree shift in frame of reference, as depicted in Figure 3.3. One can see the three core psychological needs of SDT expressed by the coach who is facilitating (supporting the coachee's needs for autonomy, competence, and relatedness) and the expert who is instructing or prescribing (operating from the medical expert role of judging, fixing, and rescuing). This shift requires a significant boost in a coach's meta-awareness to notice which role one is playing in any given moment and adjust to the optimal role for the coachee. Though it is an ongoing process for coaches, it is even more challenging for physician coaches, as the medical expert role is deeply embedded in the physician identity.

Role Model

In addition to coaches being well-equipped to apply the rich scientific foundation that supports coaching, being a role model as a coach is also vital to being an authentic inspiration to a coachee. Being a role model is particularly valuable when a physician coach is coaching a medical student or resident. Hence full engagement in working with one's own coach or self-coaching is important to a coach's impact. Coaches pursue continual cultivation of their own mindfulness, autonomy, competence, EI, psychological capital,

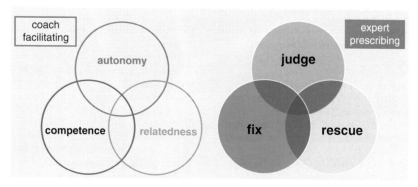

Fig. 3.3 Self-Determination Theory: Primary Human Needs.

strengths, and surfacing and outgrowing one's growth edges, areas in which coaches experience tension, doubt, stress, or strain. It's a journey that offers much meaning and nourishment to physicians as they move through the many professional phases, from student to leader.

CONCLUSION

We have covered a lot of scientific ground in this chapter to support the integrity of the coach approach and coaching competencies in medical education. We encourage readers to consider whether the definition of coaching in medical education is appropriate and complete. It is valuable for readers to explore the important theories further, identify new theories not addressed, and take time to learn from the literature along with this chapter's references and sources while practicing coaching skills. It is much easier to write about coaching than to be a competent and masterful coach. It's best not to underestimate what is needed in terms of learning, skills practice, skills evaluation, or skills assessment, and working with one's own coach. The effort to learn the coach approach is rewarded well; it's a gift to have the skills to empower others to change, grow, and thrive beyond what they can do alone.

TAKE-HOME POINTS

1. The coach approach focuses on helping coachees expand self-awareness, discover their internal values and motivation, use their strengths in new ways, and improve self-efficacy and their capacity for self-guided change of mindset and behavior.
2. It is valuable to develop and draw from a large toolbox in coaching, as each coachee and each session presents a new, unpredictable situation and an opportunity to experiment with a new tool.
3. A good coach is able to hold two mindsets at the same time—a fullness of empathy and acceptance of the coachee's situation, without judgment and criticism, along with the inspiration to help coachees to envision a better future and outgrow what is limiting their growth and potential.

QUESTIONS FOR FURTHER THOUGHT

1. What interests you most about the theories that support the coach approach?
2. How might a coach help you with your professional development, leadership, and well-being?
3. What surprises you about the coach approach?
4. What is your aspiration or vision for applying the coach approach in your work and life?

ANNOTATED BIBLIOGRAPHY

Kegan R, Lahey LL. *Immunity to change: How to overcome it and unlock potential in yourself and your organization.* Harvard Business Press; 2009.
The immunity to change model helps coaches understand the hidden forces that can block change and how to help coachees productively discover and overcome these forces.

Moore M, Tschannen-Moran B, Jackson, E. *Coaching psychology manual.* 2nd ed. Wolters Kluwer Health/Lippincott, Williams & Wilkins; 2015.
This manual is a more complete summary of many of the theories applied to coaching explored in this chapter.

Peterson C, Seligman ME. *Character strengths and virtues: A handbook and classification,* vol. 1. Oxford University Press; 2004.
This reference book is an important source of the history and science of 24 human character strengths.

Ryan R, Deci E. Chapter 20: Supporting Autonomy, Competence, and Relatedness: The Coaching Process from a Self-Determination Theory Perspective. In: English S, Sabatine JM, Brownell P, eds. *Professional coaching: Principles and practice.* 1st ed. Springer Publishing Company; 2018.
This book chapter is an overview of how coaching rests on the principles of self-determination theory, the core theory that supports the coach approach.

REFERENCES

1. Whitmore J. *Coaching for Performance: Growing Human Potential and Purpose: The Principles and Practice of Coaching and Leadership*. Hachette, UK. 2010.

2. Passmore J, Lai Yi-Ling. Coaching psychology: Exploring definitions and research contribution to practice. *Int Coaching Psychol Rev*. 2019;14(2):69–83.

3. Whitmore J. Sir John Whitmore demonstrating coaching vs instruction [Video]. *Vimeo*. https://vimeo.com/41343451. Published 2012. Accessed June 23, 2021.

4. Grant AM. Developing an agenda for teaching coaching psychology. *Int Coaching Psychol Rev*. 2011;6(1):84–99.

5. Moore M, Tschannen-Moran B, Jackson, E. *Coaching Psychology Manual*. p. 170. Wolters Kluwer Health/LWW. 2010.

6. International Coaching Federation. All Things Coaching. https://coachingfederation.org/about. Accessed June 23, 2021.

7. National Board for Health and Wellness Coaching. Health & wellness coach scope of practice. https://nbhwc.org/scope-of-practice/. Accessed June 23, 2021.

8. American Medical Association. CPT Codes. https://www.ama-assn.org/practice-management/cpt. Accessed June 23, 2021.

9. Athanasopoulou A, Dopson S. A systematic review of executive coaching outcomes: Is it the journey or the destination that matters the most? *The Leadership Quarterly*. 2018;29(1):70–88.

10. Sforzo GA, Kaye MP, Todorova I, et al. Compendium of the health and wellness coaching literature. *Am J Lifestyle Med*. 2018;12(6):436–447.

11. Sforzo GA, Kaye MP, Harenberg S, et al. Compendium of health and wellness coaching: 2019 addendum. *Am J Lifestyle Med*. 2020;14(2):155–168.

12. Schneider S, Kingsolver K, Rosdahl J. Physician coaching to enhance well-being: a qualitative analysis of a pilot intervention. *Explore*. 2014;10(6):372–379.

13. Dyrbye LN, Shanfelt TD, Gill PR, et al. Effect of a Professional Coaching Intervention on the Well-being and Distress of Physicians. A Pilot Randomized Clinical Trial. *JAMA Intern Med*. 2019;179(10):1406–1414.

14. Ryan RM, Deci EL. In Elliot AJ, ed. Brick by brick: The Origins, Development, and Future of Self-Determination Theory, vol 6, Elsevier.

15. Ryan R, Deci E. Chapter 20: Supporting Autonomy, Competence, and Relatedness: The Coaching Process from a Self-Determination Theory Perspective. In: English S, Sabatine JM, Brownell P, eds. *Professional Coaching: Principles and Practice*: Springer Publishing Company; 2018.

16. Kashdan T. *Curious? Discover the Missing Ingredient to a Fulfilling Life*: William Morrow & Co; 2019.

17. Schutte NS, Malouff JM. Increasing curiosity through autonomy of choice. *Motivation and Emotion*. 2019;43(4):563–570 2019.

18. Miller WR, Rollnick S. *Motivational Interviewing: Helping People Change*: Guilford Press; 2012.

19. Boyatzis R, Smith ML, Van Oosten E. *Helping People Change: Coaching with Compassion for Lifelong Learning and Growth*: Harvard Business Press; 2019.

20. Taylor SN, Passarelli AM, Van Oosten EB. Leadership coach effectiveness as fostering self-determined, sustained change. *The Leadership Quarterly*. 2019;30(6).

21. Moore M, Tschannen-Moran B, Jackson E. *Coaching Psychology Manual*. 2nd ed.: Wolters Kluwer Health/Lippincott, Williams & Wilkins; 2015.

22. Positive Psychology Center. University of Pennsylvania. https://ppc.sas.upenn.edu. Accessed June 23, 2021.

23. Peterson C, Seligman ME*Character Strengths and Virtues: A Handbook and Classification*, vol 1: Oxford University Press; 2004.

24. Fredrickson BL, Joiner T. Reflections on positive emotions and upward spirals. *Perspectives on Psychological Science*. 2018;13(2):194–199.

25. Luthans F, Youssef-Morgan CM. Psychological capital: An evidence-based positive approach. *Ann Rev Organizational Psychol Organizational Behav*. 2017;4:339–366.

26. Poots A, Cassidy T. Academic expectation, self-compassion, psychological capital, social support and student wellbeing. *Int J Educ Res*. 2020;99:101.

27. Whitney DD, Trosten-Bloom A. *The Power of Appreciative Inquiry: A Practical Guide to Positive Change*: Berrett-Koehler Publishers; 2010.

28. Sandars J, Murdoch-Eaton D. Appreciative inquiry in medical education. *Med Teach*. 2017;39(2):123–127.

29. David Cooperrider, PhD. Case Western Reserve University. https://weatherhead.case.edu/faculty/david-cooperrider. Accessed June 23, 2021.

30. Growth Mindset Institute. www.growthmindsetinstitute.org. Accessed July 16, 2021.

31. Kabat-Zinn J. Defining Mindfulness. Mindful.org. January 11, 2017. https://www.mindful.org/jon-kabat-zinn-defining-mindfulness/. Accessed June 23, 2021.

32. Scheepers RA, Emke H, Epstein RM, Lombarts KM. The impact of mindfulness-based interventions on doctors' well-being and performance: A systematic review. *Med Educ*. 2020;54(2):138–149.

33. Baer RA, Smith GT, Lykins E, et al. Construct validity of the five facet mindfulness questionnaire in meditating and nonmeditating samples. *Assessment*. 2008;15(3):329–342.

34. Vago DR, David SA. Self-awareness, self-regulation, and self-transcendence (S-ART): a framework for understanding the neurobiological mechanisms of mindfulness. *Front Hum Neurosci*. 2012;6:296.

35. Akrivou K, Boyatzis RE. The ideal self as the driver of intentional change. *J Manag Dev*. 2006;25(7):624–642.

36. Barrett LF. *How Emotions are Made: The Secret Life of the Brain*: Houghton Mifflin Harcourt; 2017.

37. Grewal D, Davidson HA. Emotional intelligence and graduate medical education. *JAMA*. 2008;300(10):1200–1202.

38. Neff K. Self-compassion. https://self-compassion.org/the-three-elements-of-self-compassion-2/. Accessed June 23, 2021.

39. Hayes SC. A Liberated Mind: How to Pivot Toward What Matters. *Avery*. 2020.

40. David S. Emotional Agility: Get Unstuck, Embrace Change, and Thrive in Work and Life. *Penguin*. 2016.

41. Rosenberg MB. *Nonviolent Communication: A Language of Compassion*: University of California Press; 2011.

42. Hall KL, Rossi JS. Meta-analytic examination of the strong and week principles across 48 health behaviors. *Prev Med.* 2008;46(3):266–274.

43. Prochaska JO, Velicer WF. The transtheoretical model of health behavior change. *Am J Health Promot.* 1997;12(1):38–48.

44. Nowack K. Facilitating successful behavior change: Beyond goal setting to goal flourishing. *Consult Psychol J Pract Res.* 2017;69(3):153.

45. Oettingen G. Rethinking positive thinking: Inside the new science of motivation. *Current.* 2015.

46. Saddawi-Konefka D, Baker K, Guarino A, et al. Changing resident physician studying behaviors: A randomized, comparative effectiveness trial of goal setting versus use of WOOP. *J Grad Med Educ.* 2017;9(4):451.

47. Clancy AL, Binkert J. *Pivoting: A Coach's Guide to Igniting Substantial Change*: Springer; 2016.

48. Snyder CR, Harris C, Anderson JR, et al. The will and the ways: development and validation of an individual-differences measure of hope. *J Pers Soc Psychol.* 1991;60(4):570–585.

49. Neenan M, Palmer S, eds. *Cognitive Behavioural Coaching in Practice: An Evidence Based Approach*: Routledge; 2013.

50. Neenan M. Using Socratic questioning in coaching. *J Ration-Emot Cogn-Behav Ther.* 2009;27(4):249–264.

51. Kegan R. *In Over Our Heads: The Mental Demands of Modern Life*: Harvard University Press; 1994.

52. Kegan R, Lahey LL. *Immunity to Change: How to Overcome It and Unlock Potential in Yourself and Your Organization*: Harvard Business Press; 2009.

4

Competencies for Academic Coaches

Kendra Parekh, Sherilyn Smith, and Simran Singh

LEARNING OBJECTIVES

1. Discuss the need for coaching competencies.
2. Describe the skills and competencies required for successful coaching.

3. Outline specific observable behaviors that demonstrate coaching competencies.

CHAPTER OUTLINE

CHAPTER SUMMARY

In this chapter, we highlight the core competencies essential to academic coaching in medical education and describe coaching competencies as they relate to academic coaching in medical education across the continuum of learners. We discuss the need for coaching competencies to drive coach development, program evaluation, and desired coaching outcomes and summarize the current frameworks of coaching competencies. Last, we delineate specific observable coaching behaviors that demonstrate coaching competence.

OVERVIEW OF COACHING COMPETENCIES

With medical education shifting to competency-based medical education (CBME), educators are adopting the principles of coaching as a method to individualize education and support each learner in their development of the necessary competencies and skills for successful career progression.[1] Coaches help learners to review performance data, identify gaps, create goals, develop plans to manage existing and potential challenges, improve performance, and further professional identity and leadership development. Coaching encourages learners to become competent, reflective physicians and master adaptive learners.

As coaching continues to grow and evolve in CBME systems, there is a concomitant need to ensure appropriate development of and support for educators as coaches.[2] The coaching role is new to the majority of medical educators and requires a new set of skills and competencies that educators must develop to be effective coaches.[3] Clearly articulated coaching competencies in the context of medical education are a necessary step on this journey.

Whereas coaching competencies have been created for professional executive and health and wellness coaches, coaching competencies designed for medical educators are only beginning to emerge.[4-7] Well-articulated coaching competencies are necessary to support the development of educators as coaches in medical education, as competencies help educators understand what is expected of the coaching role and what successful coaching looks like and help drive program outcomes. Coaching competencies can be used to assess coach performance and conduct coaching program evaluation.[8] Coaching competencies support a shared mental model of coaching in medical education and can

Vignette

Lisa is the director of her medical school's longitudinal coaching and professional development program for medical students. Each coach is assigned four students per academic year. She is reviewing student feedback regarding faculty coaches and notices that Darren has significantly lower ratings than all other faculty coaches. He has been a faculty member in the coaching program for a little more than 1 year and has won teaching awards from students and residents at his previous institution. The coaching program has a well-established onboarding program and a collaborative community of practice among the coaches.

Thought Questions

1. What information would be helpful for Lisa to gather as she explores the student feedback with Darren?
2. Considering the coaching competencies, what skills and strategies might Lisa use when talking with Darren?
3. What coaching resources or tools can Lisa provide to Darren?

help advance research on coaching. Ultimately, coaching competencies may inform learner outcomes, institutional culture, and patient or other health care–related outcomes.

Professional coaching organizations have translated a variety of theoretical frameworks into science-based coaching competencies. Table 4.1 compares the competencies from several major professional coaching organizations. All organizations have competencies in professionalism or ethics that include the explicit requirement of creating a coaching agreement.[4-7] All have multiple competencies around trust, relationship building, and communication skills.[4-7] Finally, a subset (business and wellness) have specific requirements around contextual knowledge that is ideally leveraged during coaching practice.[6-7]

The shared professional coaching competencies are highly applicable to academic coaching in medical education. Professional standards articulated by these organizations align with the fiduciary responsibilities of physicians, and many aspects of the communication competencies align with those that are valuable in patient-centered care approaches. A subset of professional coaching organizations has specific knowledge for practice competencies, like the knowledge for practice requirements in medicine. All coaching organizations value professional development

TABLE 4.1	Comparison of Professional Coaching Competencies			
Competency	Association for Coaching	International Coaching Federation	Worldwide Association of Business Coaches	National Board for Health & Wellness Coaching
Professional conduct	X	X	X	X
Coaching agreement	X	X	X	X
Ethics	X	X	X	X
Legal	X	X	X	X
Trust-based relationship	X	X	X	X
Supportive presence	X	X	X	X
Active listening	X	X	X	X
Questioning	X	X	X	X
Create awareness	X	X	X	X
Communicate clearly	X		X	
Develop actions, goals, planning	X	X	X	X
Accountability, managing process	X	X	X	X
Knowledge[a]	X		X	X
Professional development	X	X	X	X

[a]Knowledge: business content—entrepreneurial knowledge, skills, attitudes; business knowledge, systems thinking, organizational change, behavior, development principles; leadership issues; facility with assessment tools & strategies for business coaches; health and wellness content—health promotion, chronic disease, health behaviors, social and behavior risk factors; positive psychology.

and have requirements for continuing education to maintain certification similar to the norms for the medical profession.

Academic coaching competencies for medical education have been developed and fall into five broad categories: coaching structure and process; relational skills; coaching skills; coaching theories and models; and coach development. Table 4.2 outlines competencies for coaching in medical education.[9] Using the master adaptive learner (MAL) framework to scaffold academic coaching leverages adult learning theory and self-determination theory in a familiar pattern of continuous quality improvement used in improvement science.[10]

COACHING COMPETENCIES IN ACTION

As we seek to develop competencies in coaches, it is important to understand what the competencies can look like in practice. We discuss each category of coaching competencies and behaviors that may be reported or observed.

TABLE 4.2 Coaching Competencies for Medical Education

Competency Domain	Observed Behaviors and Actions
Coaching Structure and Process	
Establish coaching agreement	In orientation session, explore and align on: • Role of coach (facilitator, not mentor or instructor) and coachee (ready to commit to self-discovery, change) • Coaching program principles (confidentiality; expectations; number, duration, and timing of sessions; email/phone communication; program length, etc.) • Coachee's needs and interests (e.g., well-being, resilience, stress, communication, academic performance, professional development) • General outline of coachee's coaching goals or outcomes (how will we know the coaching program was successful?) • Use of assessments and homework assignments for self-awareness and progress or outcomes measurement • Support of authentic feedback from coach to coachee and learner to coach; continually evaluate coach/learner fit
Manage coaching sessions	• Schedule sessions (e.g., 30–60 mins every 2–4 weeks for 3 months) • Initial sessions—debrief assessments; support coachee in developing vision or goals; explore values, motivation, strengths, and action plan • Ongoing sessions—coachee identifies area for exploration, explores coachee progress and learning, cultivates self-awareness with growth mindset, updates action plan • Coach documents notes as needed • Closing session—harvest progress and learning, and explore coachee's next steps without coach
Manage process and accountability	• Help coachee integrate the Master Adaptive Learner model, including planning, learning, assessing, and adjusting • Help coachee design accountability practices (e.g., check-ins, progress notes, or coaching journal) • Support coachee in tracking progress (progress notes, 0–10 rulers, graphs, apps) • Hold coachee accountable for commitments, session attendance, engagement, and progress • Explore how coaching relationship is working and not working, how to improve • Discern whether coachee would benefit more from a teaching, mentoring, or counseling role

Continued

TABLE 4.2   Coaching Competencies for Medical Education—cont'd

Competency Domain	Observed Behaviors and Actions
Relational Skills	
Establish a meaningful coaching relationship	• Establish trust and mutual respect • Demonstrate honesty and integrity • Use nonjudgmental and accepting communication, unconditional regard, to create psychological safety (to explore challenges and feedback) • Appreciate and accept diversity of coachee values, goals, perspectives • Address and resolve discord with coachee
Use coaching communication	Elicit self-awareness, meta-awareness, self-reflection, progress: • Be present and give undivided attention • Engage in open, curious inquiry with no agenda or judgment • Use active listening (listen fully to words, thoughts, emotions, meaning, what's not being said, coachee's frame of reference) • Engage in reflections (e.g., summaries, amplified, empathy) • Use affirmation; reflect strengths, progress, successes, and learning
Cultivate coachee's emotional intelligence	Help coachee navigate emotional states and emotional well-being: • Help coachee cultivate positive emotions (positive questions) • Help coachee cultivate mindfulness and improve emotional awareness, meta-awareness • Help coachee cultivate self-compassion • Help coachee process emotions—noticing, naming, and experiencing • Help coachee explore and leverage emotions as growth opportunities—what needs are not met, what would help meet those needs • Help coachee cultivate self-regulation, recognizing emotions are produced by the brain based on past experiences, not present reality
Coaching Skills	
Support coachee in being a master adaptive learner	• Help coachee understand their abilities in the master adaptive learner cycle (planning, learning, assessing, adjusting) • Support and guide coachee in engagement in being a master adaptive learner (critical thinking, reflection, self-monitoring, metacognition)
Support coachee in cultivating well-being and professional fulfillment	• Use open inquiry to support coachee in defining a vision of ideal self or goals for optimum well-being and professional fulfillment
Support coachee in improving motivation and self-efficacy	• Support coachees in cultivating key characteristics to the master adaptive learning process—curiosity about learning, intrinsic motivation, growth mindset, and resilience • Explore coachee's personal values and how they are expressed in vision, goals, and action plans • Cultivate coachee's internal motivation for change, including meaning, purpose, or calling • Explore coachee strengths • Explore coachee's resources and psychological capital (hope, optimism, self-efficacy, and resilience)
Help coachee overcome challenges with cocreative collaboration	• Support coachee in problem-solving and cocreative brainstorming on new perspectives and possibilities • Support coachee in processing feedback • Continue to elicit MAL characteristics—curiosity about learning, intrinsic motivation, growth mindset, and resilience

TABLE 4.2 **Coaching Competencies for Medical Education—cont'd**	
Competency Domain	**Observed Behaviors and Actions**
Coaching Theories and Models	
Identify and use coaching theories and tools that best fit coachee's needs	• Identify and use the most appropriate coaching theories and tools best suited to the coachee's needs and goals
Use flexibility and adaptability	• Discern the changing (evolving) needs of the coachee and choose the appropriate inquiry, model, or tool to support the coachee in achieving desired goals • Identify how the differences in goals may affect the utility of previously used coaching models and tools
Coach Development	
Cultivate self-development	• Seek coach training and ongoing coaching education • Work with a professional coach for self-development • Ensure own work is consistent with national standards
Cultivate self-management	• Hold self accountable to using coaching skills and processes, mindfully noticing and shifting when advising or mentoring • Cultivate own well-being as a role model—autonomy, competence, mindfulness, emotional intelligence, positivity, strengths, growth
Recognize limitations	• Recognize limitations as a coach and when to refer to counseling or other specialized services • Recognize good coach/coachee fit • Recognize when coaching might need to come to an end and facilitate this transition

Adapted from Wolff M, Deiorio NM, Juve AM, et al. Beyond advising and mentoring: competencies for coaching in medical education. *Med Teach.* 2021;43(10):1210–1213.

Coaching Structure and Process

The first category is the coaching structure and process. It is important for the coach and coachee to have a coaching agreement so that each party has a clear understanding of what the goals and objectives are for the process and the limitations of the coaching relationship. The initial coaching session can serve as an orientation to the coaching process and include a discussion of the role of the coach and coachee; coaching program principles; and the coachee's needs, interests, and coaching goals. The coach may wish to discuss the use of self-assessment tools such as the VIA Character Strengths Survey or the Professional Fulfillment Inventory[11] and the use of homework assignments to promote self-awareness as well as the progress and outcome measures that may be used. From the onset of the coaching relationship, both the coach and coachee will benefit from a commitment to providing authentic feedback to continually evaluate the fit of the coaching relationship. Coaching agreements can be standardized within a coaching program and individualized to learner needs. An example of coaching agreements is shown in Fig. 4.1.

When managing sessions, coaches empower coachees to set the agenda for the session in order to harness coachees' internal values and motivation, in alignment with self-determination theory.[12] Initial coaching sessions can be used to debrief any completed self-assessments; support the coachee in developing goals using tools such as wish, outcome, obstacle, plan (WOOP) and specific, measurable, achievable, relevant, time-based (SMART) goals; and exploring values, motivation, and strengths to develop action plans. Ongoing sessions may focus on a coachee's identified areas for exploration, review of progress, and continued cultivation of self-awareness. Through the coaching relationship, the coach supports the coachee's integration of the MAL model, including exploration of the planning, learning, assessing, and adjusting phases. The coach's documentation of coaching sessions includes clear expectations that are transparent to the coachee, including what is documented and who will have access to the documentation. Coaches monitor the coachee's progress and hold the coachee accountable, using a myriad of relational and communication skills. Similarly, coaches self-monitor

Example of portfolio coaching contract
Oregon Health & Science University

Portfolio coach program

The Colleges program was begun in 2012 with the core mission of inspiring and supporting students in defining and reaching their full potential. Portfolio Coaches listen to students' reflections upon their educational experiences in order to improve performance. They assist students in creating and meeting academic goals.

Coach and student relationship

The coaching relationship requires active participation and commitment of both coach and student. As such, it is important to note the following:

- The relationship will change and develop over time, with ongoing discussion of coaching relationship and roles.
- Continuity of coaching pairs and meetings over the course of medical school is important.
- Trust is a core element of the relationship.
- Confidentiality is essential. The coach will not be involved in student grading or evaluation, including clinical rotations. Coaches cannot be made to reveal any information shared in a coaching session unless the student is in danger.

Academic coaching agreement and expectations

Student expectations

- Be open and honest with coach, including strengths, limitations, and challenges
- Be open to feedback
- Come to scheduled meetings on time and contact coach in advance with any potential schedule conflicts
- Come to meeting with an agenda: academics, wellness, academic and career goals, outside concerns, expectations
- Help coach define optimal ways to assist you
- Respond to coach communications in a timely manner
- Inform coach of any relevant problems or challenges (academic, personal or other) in a timely manner
- Support other members of cohort - in same class and other classes
- Follow through with mutually agreed upon plans/action items

Coach expectations

- Respond to student concerns in a timely manner
- Clarify desired methods of communication with student: email, text, etc.
- Review student evaluations and grades prior to meetings and identify areas of concern
- Follow up with prior concerns and action items
- Effectively document coaching sessions to assist with student growth, while maintaining appropriate confidentiality
- As needed, refer student to appropriate resources

_____   _____   _____
Student   Coach   Date

Fig. 4.1 Example of a portfolio coaching contract.

and hold themselves accountable to the coach approach in the coaching relationship. Coaches understand the limits of the coaching relationship such as when it is appropriate to recommend counseling or other specialized services (e.g., assessment for learning disabilities) or when to end the coaching relationship. In a closing session, the coach can help the coachee explore the next steps without a coach and support future planning. Medical educators are often called upon to serve multiple roles, including as advisers and mentors. Educators serving in the role of coach are vigilant and recognize when they have moved out of the coaching role and are providing advice or offering solutions to their coachee before fully exploring and brainstorming on the coachee's ideas and options. The following is an example of a competent coach engaged in the coaching process and structure.

This is the first session with the coachee. The coach has prepared for the session and feels ready to meet the coachee. The coach opens the session with an introduction and invites the coachee to introduce herself and discuss her reasons for seeking a coach. After actively listening, the coach explores the coaching agreement, and the coach and coachee finalize the agreement to the satisfaction of both parties. The coach keeps brief notes from the session along with the coaching agreement. In subsequent sessions, the coach continually checks in with the coachee at the start of the session and invites the coachee to set the session agenda. The coach uses open-ended questions to probe progress on goal achievement, focusing first on what went well and harvesting what has been learned in order to increase self-awareness of positive resources.

At one point, the coachee shares her experience of heightened anxiety and stress. Although the coach is capable of providing teaching on relaxation techniques and anxiety management, the coach initiates a brainstorming conversation on possible techniques and mindsets that would be helpful. The coach then recognizes that the anxiety level experienced by the coachee may be at a clinical level and suggests a referral for therapeutic support. The coachee agrees to the referral, preserving the coaching focus on coachee autonomy and goals and not on clinical management. The coaching relationship grows stronger, and the coachee continues to progress well toward her goals, while separately getting clinical support for anxiety.

Relational Skills

The next category of coaching competencies is relational skills. The entire foundation of coaching is built on the relationship between the coach and coachee, paramount to growth and positive outcomes. Coaches establish meaningful coaching relationships and demonstrate emotional intelligence (exploring and clarifying the coachee's emotional states), adaptability (changing direction when needed), and effective communication (succinct, open, and affirming questions and reflections).

The establishment of meaningful relationships includes developing and maintaining trust with the coachee and creating a climate of mutual respect and safety by using nonjudgmental communications while appreciating the coachee's diverse experiences and perspectives. Coaches demonstrate honesty and integrity. Perhaps most importantly, coaches show unconditional positive regard for the coachees and their strengths and inner resourcefulness. This creates psychological safety, allowing for further exploration of challenges and feedback. Coaches will use coaching communication that includes being present with the coachee and providing undivided attention and active listening. To build the coaching relationship further, coaches continue to notice, respond to, and empathize with the coachee's emotional states, inviting self-awareness and deepening self-reflection. Effective communication is demonstrated by actively listening without expressing opinions or judgment and asking powerful, open questions that expand horizons and self-reflection. A coach is flexible and adaptable in using different techniques as called for by the coachee's situation.

Coaches cultivate a coachee's emotional intelligence; this includes helping the coachee navigate emotional states and emotional well-being (see Chapter 3 sections on positive psychology and emotional intelligence).[13] There are multiple ways for coaches to demonstrate competence in this area. Coaches can help coachees cultivate positive emotions, mindfulness, and self-compassion. They can help the coachee process emotions and leverage emotions for growth opportunities. These interactions further develop a coachee's self-regulation. Next is an example of a competent coach using relational skills.

The coach has just finished a morning of clinic and has a full afternoon of coaching sessions. When the coach looks at the schedule, they realize that one of their more challenging coachees is first on the list. Recognizing their own feelings, the coach takes a few moments to do a deep breathing exercise and calls to mind why they chose to become a coach in the first place. The coachee arrives for the session. The coach warmly greets the coachee and checks in with them. The coach asks an open question: "What stands out for you as you reflect on your goals for the last week?" When the coachee doesn't provide many details, the coach shifts the inquiry to "Tell me about something that went well for you in the last week?" followed by silence and reflections to further ignite the conversation. After the session concludes, the coach takes a few moments to reflect on the session and consider other lines of inquiry they could use when coachees aren't being engaged. The coach then does some brief movements and deep breathing to prepare for the next session.

Coaching Skills

One coaching skill that is especially relevant in medical education is to support the development of MALs. The MAL is a conceptual model that proposes a cycle of planning, learning, assessing, and adjusting that supports the development of lifelong learning and adaptive expertise.[10,14] Coaches are able to describe and discuss the MAL model to help coachees choose to develop into adaptive learners.[14] Coaches also facilitate conversations that help coachees improve well-being and professional growth and fulfillment. The coachee is the expert on themselves, and coaches use their relational skills to fully understand what well-being and professional fulfillment look like for each coachee.

Although it may be tempting to provide advice to the coachee (particularly if they are a more junior learner) or to fill in knowledge deficits, coaches maintain their coaching role and support coachee autonomy, motivation, and self-determination. The greater the expertise of the coach in the coachee's chosen areas of development, the more difficult this may be. Coaches support coachees in developing well-being and professional fulfillment through supporting the coachee in the development of a vision of the ideal self or goals for optimum well-being and professional fulfillment. Coaches remember to be creative with open questions and perceptive reflections and other tools to support the coachee to expand perspectives and possibilities and enable growth.[15,16] Coachees are the driver of their own growth; if a coach pushes for growth, coachees can respond by resisting or complying rather than making choices that are based on their own interests and values. Coaches work in partnership with coachees, and the coachee feels empowered to set the agenda and express their values and needs.

Through supporting the coachee in improving motivation and self-efficacy, coaches can promote key drivers of the master adaptive learning process, including curiosity about learning, intrinsic motivation, growth mindset, and resilience (see Chapter 2). Coaches are mindful to use language, processes, and skills that increase coachee's intrinsic motivation for change and capitalize on the coachee's strengths. Utilization of strength assessments can be helpful in this process. They can also draw out coachee's psychological capital (e.g., hope, optimism, self-efficacy, etc.). Coaches help coachees overcome challenges with cocreative collaboration and support coachees in problem-solving and cocreative brainstorming on new perspectives and possibilities. Coaches help a coachee process feedback; this is an opportunity to help the coachee continue to develop characteristics of master adaptive learners and reframe feedback as learning opportunities and opportunities for growth. Next is an example of a competent coach using coaching skills.

In preparation for their upcoming session, the coach reviewed notes from prior sessions and wanted to follow up on a few things. When the coachee arrives for the session, they appear distracted and disengaged. Recognizing this, the coach notes the coachee's current state warmly and empathetically, without judgment. The coachee discloses that they received a poor grade on an exam and have "felt lost" in their small group learning sessions. The coach prioritizes the coachee's need at this moment over the coach's agenda and uses open-ended questions to probe further into the coachee's situation. Using the MAL model, the coach helps the coachee discover that they have not been using effective learning strategies to study for exams. Subsequently, the coachee sets a goal to talk with their course directors about learning strategies and a plan to monitor their learning. The coach and coachee review the coachee's strengths and discuss how these strengths can be used to support the implementation of any recommended learning strategies. The coachee leaves the session feeling empowered and confident that they can implement the strategies and can improve their grade and small group performance.

Coaching Theories and Models

As noted earlier, coaches are adaptable and have a variety of skills and tools to use during coaching sessions. This requires coaches to stay up to date on coaching models and tools to support learning—modeling the master adaptive learner. Coaches acquire new skills and tools as their coaching experience grows. They will simultaneously need to develop judgment and decision-making skills to select the most appropriate coaching model or coaching skills to apply to the situation at hand. Coaches themselves can benefit from coachee feedback, mentor coaching, and developmental coaching. Additionally, coaches remain cognizant of the fact that the coachee will grow and change as the relationship progresses. Coaches are alert to these changing needs and adjust coaching sessions accordingly. The coaching process is dynamic. Coaching does not continue indefinitely, although coaching relationships may continue for many years. In line with self-determination theory, coaches support a coachee's autonomy and over time, there may be less need for coaching or fewer items on the coachee's initial agenda. In response, the coaching process and structure may end or evolve to explore new growth topics.

Coach Development

As noted previously, coaching organizations value professional development as an integral part of coaching. Thus coaches engage in continual development. Coaches seek additional training and professional development opportunities. They may also work with a professional coach for further self-development. Although there are currently no national standards for coaching in medical education, coaches can continually seek out training opportunities and build community among academic coaches to support coach development and accountability. Coaches work to cultivate self-management, using mindfulness techniques to hold themselves accountable for using coaching skills and processes and noticing when they are advising or mentoring. As coaches are supporting coachees in developing their well-being, coaches are mindful of cultivating their own well-being and serving as a role model for the coachee. Last, a coach recognizes the limitations of coaching and refers coachees for additional support when necessary. As discussed previously, the coach will also monitor the coaching relationship, recognizing when the relationship is not optimal and when coaching might need to come to an end. Next is an example of a competent coach engaging in coach development.

After coaching for approximately 1 year, the coach deliberately plans time to reflect on their first year of coaching. Guided by this reflection the coach makes a plan for self-development, including a list of coach development sessions to attend. The coach specifically noticed that they tend to provide advice, particularly to early learners who are struggling with common problems. Recognizing this, the coach actively seeks out coaching from an experienced colleague. Additionally, the coach has brainstormed ways to support their own well-being and is planning to attend an upcoming mindfulness training offered by their institution. The coach writes out their goals for their coaching along with their development plan and schedules time for reflection over the coming months to track their progress.

ASSESSMENT OF COACHING COMPETENCY

As we seek to advance coaching competencies in academic coaching, we can consider the core components of CBME as developed by Van Melle et al. and use this as a framework to advance coaching competencies.[17] CBME systems are focused on outcomes and clearly explicate desired outcomes. There is a progressive sequencing of competencies with learning experiences and teaching tailored to the competencies. Programmatic assessment is essential and emphasizes personalized, actionable feedback. The coaching competencies discussed in this chapter are a first step in this process as they describe the desired actions and outcomes of a competent coach. As institutions and organizations seek to use these competencies, they should give

consideration to the sequencing of them and deliberately develop teaching activities for each competency. Coaches should have the opportunity to participate in learning experiences designed to support competency development. Instrumental in this process is feedback to coaches and programmatic evaluation of coaching programs.

Although research is only beginning to emerge on assessing coaching competency, the same assessment methods we employ in medical education can be used to assess coaching competencies. Foundational knowledge can be assessed with tests whether constructed or selected response. Simulation is a viable option to assess relational, communication, and coaching skills. Direct observation by peers, trainers, or mentor coaches is also an available assessment method. Coach self-report and self-assessment could be used to assess emotional intelligence and other competencies. Self-assessment has the added benefit of simultaneously helping coaches develop their skills in self-monitoring. Evaluations from coachees could also be used to assess the relational, communication, and coaching skills of the coach.[18] Regardless of the assessment method chosen, it will be essential to be thoughtful and deliberate in the design of assessments and in the development of programmatic assessment of coaches and coaching programs. The coaching relationship should not be disrupted, and the program of coach assessment must support coaches and be conducted in the spirit of coaching.

CONCLUSION

Coaching competencies in medical education are similar to other professional coaching competencies, although specific to the context of medicine and medical education. Well-articulated competencies are necessary to advance coaching across the continuum of medical education and provide clear expectations of coaches. Coaching competencies in medical education are divided into four categories (coaching process and structure, relational skills, coaching skills, and coaching theories and research) each with its own set of observable and learnable behaviors.

TAKE-HOME POINTS

1. Coaching competencies in medical education are necessary to support the development of medical educators as coaches and to develop a shared mental model of coaching in medical education, to evaluate coach and program outcomes, and to advance research.
2. Self-determination theory is a robust, core underlying theory for all coaching.

3. Coaching competencies in medical education can be divided into five categories: coaching process and structure, relational skills, coaching skills, coaching theories and models, and coach development.
4. Coaching competencies can be taught and developed through training and practice.

QUESTIONS FOR FURTHER THOUGHT

1. How will you incorporate the coaching competencies into faculty development programs or coaching program development?
2. When training new coaches, which competencies might be particularly challenging for new coaches to navigate? How will you support the development of these competencies?
3. How will you assess the development of coaching competencies in your coaches?
4. What approaches would you use if one of your coaches was having difficulties with competency development?

ANNOTATED BIBLIOGRAPHY

Association for Coaching. AC Coaching Competencies Framework. https://cdn.ymaws.com/www.associationforcoaching.com/resource/resmgr/Accreditation/Accred_General/Coaching_Competency_Framewor.pdf. Accessed July 26, 2021.
Provides a detailed set of competencies for coaches and executive coaches.

Brooks JV, Istas K, Barth BE. Becoming a coach: experiences of faculty educators learning to coach medical students. *BMC Med Educ.* 2020;20:208.
A qualitative study of faculty at a single medical school that describes the process of faculty becoming coaches, including the benefits and challenges of being a coach.

Deiorio NM, Carney PA, Kahl LE, Juve AM. Coaching: a new model for academic and career achievement. *Med Educ Online.* 2016;21(1):1087–2981.
Provides a definition of coaching and core constructs pertinent to coaching in medical education.

International Coach Federation. ICF core competencies. https://coachfederation.org/core-competencies. Accessed April 1, 2020.
Provides a detailed set of competencies used in professional coaching.

National Board of Medical Examiners and National Board for Health and Wellness Coaching. Health and wellness coach certifying exam: content outline with resources. https://www.nbme.org/sites/default/files/2020-06/HWCCE_Content_Outline_with_Resources_2020.pdf. Published June 2020. Accessed July 26, 2021.
Provides a detailed set of competencies specific for health and wellness coaches.

REFERENCES

1. Deiorio NM, Carney PA, Kahl LE, Juve AM. Coaching: a new model for academic and career achievement. *Med Educ Online.* 2016;21(1):1087–2981.
2. Orr CJ, Sonnadara RR. Coaching by design: exploring a new approach to faculty development in a competency-based medical education curriculum. *Adv Med Educ Prac.* 2019;10:229–244.
3. Brooks JV, Istas K, Barth BE. Becoming a coach: experiences of faculty educators learning to coach medical students. *BMC Med Educ.* 2020;20:208.
4. Association of Coaching. AC Coaching Competencies Framework. https://cdn.ymaws.com/www.associationforcoaching.com/resource/resmgr/Accreditation/Accred_General/Coaching_Competency_Framewor.pdf. Accessed July 26, 2021.
5. International Coach Federation. ICF core competencies. https://coachfederation.org/core-competencies. Accessed July 26, 2021.
6. Worldwide Association of Business Coaches. Business coaching competencies. https://www.wabccoaches.com/includes/popups/competencies.html. Accessed July 26, 2021.
7. National Board of Medical Examiners and National Board for Health and Wellness Coaching. Health and wellness coach certifying exam: content outline with resources. https://www.nbme.org/sites/default/files/2020-06/HWCCE_Content_Outline_with_Resources_2020.pdf. Published June 2020. Accessed July 26, 2021.
8. Carney PA, Bonura EM, Kraakevik JA, et al. Measuring coaching in undergraduate medical education: the development and psychometric validation of new instruments. *J Gen Intern Med.* 2019;34(5):677–683.
9. Wolff M, Deiorio N, Juve AM, et al. Beyond advising and mentoring: competencies for coaching in medical education. *Med Teach.* 2021;43(10):1210–1213.
10. Cutrer WB, Miller B, Pusic MV, et al. Fostering the development of Master Adaptive Learners: A conceptual model to guide skill acquisition in medical education. *Acad Med.* 2017;92(1):70–74.
11. VIA Institute on Character. https://www.viacharacter.org. Accessed July 26, 2021.
12. Ryan RM, Deci EL. Supporting autonomy, competence and relatedness: The coaching process from a self-determination theory perspective. In: English S, Sabatine JM, Brownell P, eds. *Professional Coaching: Principles and Practice.* New York, NY: Springer; 2018:231–247.
13. Kauffman C. Positive psychology: The science at the heart of coaching. In: Stober DR, Grant AM, eds. *Evidence Based Coaching Handbook: Putting Best Practices to Work for Your Clients.* Hoboken, NJ: Wiley; 2006:219-253.
14. Deiorio NM, Juve AM. How can I best support master adaptive learners using coaching. In: Cutrer WB, Pusic MV,

Gruppen LD, Hammoud MM, Santen SS, eds. *The Master Adaptive Learner*. Philadelphia: Elsevier; 2020:125–137.

15. Neenan M, Dryden W. *Life Coaching: A Cognitive-behavioural Approach*. East Sussex, NY: Brunner-Routledge; 2002.

16. Ives Y. What is 'coaching'? An exploration of conflicting paradigms. *Int J Evid Based Coach Ment*. 2008;6(2):100–113.

17. Van Melle E, Frank JR, Holmboe ES, et al. A core components framework for evaluating implementation of competency-based medical education programs. *Acad Med*. 2019;94(7):1002–1009.

18. Carney PA, Bonura EM, Kraakevik JA, et al. Measuring coaching in undergraduate medical education: the development and psychometric validation of new instruments. *J Gen Intern Med*. 2019;34(5):677–683.

5

Overview of Individual, Team, and Peer Coaching

Christine Thatcher, Kurt Pfeifer, J. Aaron Allgood, and M. Melinda Sanders

LEARNING OBJECTIVES

1. Define types of coaching, including individual, team, group, and peer coaching.
2. Identify the essential components of a coaching session.
3. Analyze and adapt to individual settings using suggested tools for success.

CHAPTER OUTLINE

CHAPTER SUMMARY

We designed this chapter for the new and experienced coach alike. We cover information on the role of the coach and different types of structures, approaches, and expectations in order to provide a foundation to the role. Program differences and institutional culture create variations in the setting, but the central theme of supporting learners in their goals and their development is a mainstay of any coaching program. Although our focus here is on medical student and resident coaching, lessons learned are transferable to other educational settings.

INTRODUCTION

The role of academic coach is a rewarding experience for both the coach and the coachee. These rewards are realized through a relationship built upon trust; meaningful exchange driven by the learner; reflective listening; and asking appropriate, open-ended questions. The setting, expectations, and developmental stage of the learner contribute to the strategy a coach may enlist to support the learner's trajectory toward their personal and professional goals. The focus of this chapter is to prepare the coach by considering different types of coaching and approaches. This chapter also provides a compendium of tips for success.

Coaching is similar but different from mentoring and advising. Although these constructs overlap, it is important to distinguish the charge or role of the coach. Coaching focuses on understanding where someone is at a certain moment in time related to their skills, training, and goals and where they would like to be holistically in the near and long-term future. An overall assessment of well-being is a critical component to helping the individual plan for progress toward their goals, thus creating a relationship of trust, which is essential to make goal setting and planning effective. The coach guides by establishing a trusting relationship, actively listening, asking clarifying questions, and thus helping the learner rise to the occasion and meet milestones in their education through a nonjudgmental approach. Students and residents increasingly take responsibility for their learning and growth of their professional identity, as well as for developing healthy habits of reflection and well-being as a result of this coaching effort. For a complete exploration of the competencies involved in coaching, see Chapter 4.

Coaching does not come naturally to many, and a structured approach for newer coaches with support through faculty development provides the underpinning to maintain the budding relationship. Coaching peers creates a support system for sharing experiences and learning from each other. For both faculty- and peer-led coaching, activities can be conducted one-on-one or in group settings. This chapter provides the scaffolding for coaches at any stage of their involvement and advice for program leadership in an effort to prepare coaches for successful encounters in individual and group settings.

TYPES OF COACHING PROGRAMS

Coaching programs have many similarities across the spectrum but will often differ in focus. The programmatic differences are institution specific and driven by the culture and needs of that institution. The multiple program goals range in emphasis but collectively have the same definition of coaching in mind. A review of the literature on coaching in medical education identifies common coaching motivations, such as well-being, resilience, and stress reduction, whereas other programs focus on professional development through positive feedback. Alternatively, coaching programs may focus on improving nontechnical skills. Such programs work to improve teamwork, enhance decision-making skills, and improve communication skills. Other programs focus on technical skills, such as those aimed at improving surgical skills in a simulated setting.[1] Whether focused on technical or nontechnical skills, many coaching programs are structured to facilitate progression of learners through their academic competencies or milestones. This coaching can be based on directly observed behaviors, on reviewing assessments, and/or on self-reported behaviors and attitudes.

In this chapter we discuss coaching in several formats: individual (one-on-one), team coaching, group coaching, and peer or near-peer coaching. Coaching programs vary in length but usually involve a longitudinal relationship. This concept of longevity is important to consider and goes hand-in-hand with planning.

Individual coaching is based on relationship building between the coach and the learner. Although the coach may be assigned a group of learners, they work with each as an individual and build trust over time. This type of coaching is used broadly for both medical students and residents. Coaches review the learner's personal and professional goals and provide support for professional development. As faculty coaches in most programs have several learners at the same academic level, group activities may help support peer-to-peer connections within the group.

Team coaching focuses on collective goal setting for a team and exploring with the members opportunities to become more effective. In the health professions, effective teamwork is important throughout training and in the clinical setting. An example of team coaching from the nursing education literature uses a gap analysis filled out by each team member prior to the coaching session.[2] The session opens with a review and clarification of team goals and objectives followed by a review of the gap analysis provided by the coach. The team members share their responses to that analysis and then share what each member observed and learned about their team experience. They then identify strengths the team can leverage to develop together. The team then outlines their primary and secondary goals and action plans to move forward. Developing high-performance teams is widely used across both business and health care to solve problems and carry out ongoing quality improvement.

Team coaching is also highly applicable to medical education. For example, team-based learning (TBL) is a broadly used pedagogy and creates teams that learn to work together for problem-solving and support. Coaches can coach a TBL team on their learning process and also help them as they learn to provide and receive peer feedback.[3]

Vignette 1

Sam, a first-year medical student, is having difficulty transitioning into medical school and is really struggling with the workload and isolation from friends and family. She is experiencing impostor syndrome as she navigates her first few months. Sam met her coach during orientation but has since entrenched herself in her studies and does not think to reach out to her coach. Many weeks go by, and Sam slips deeper into isolation. Her scores are within the average of the class, so she is not raising any red flags to her course directors and deans.

Thought Questions
1. How can a coaching program help Sam become more successful?
2. In what ways can the coach engage Sam early on to build trust and offer value through the coaching process?

Group coaching is an attractive format for coaching programs because it can more efficiently cover universally important topics. Examples of such content include mindfulness exercises, diversity/inclusion, and leadership/communication skills.[4] Additionally, group coaching sessions enhance community building and peer support. Group meetings allow for highlighting the strengths of individual members, thus increasing learners' respect for others as well as their sense of self-efficacy.

Optimal group coaching requires several unique considerations (Table 5.1). First, coaches should understand that individuals in the group may have shared goals (successful completion of medical school or residency), and the program may be using group coaching to achieve generalized objectives, but learners also bring their unique expectations and needs. When paired with one-on-one coaching, coaches can develop an understanding of each learner's specific perspectives and needs and factor these into group meetings. Even if a coach is only engaged in group coaching, it may be beneficial for them to meet at least once with individual members to develop rapport and understand expectations. Structuring group coaching meetings to allow time for "checking in" and sharing individual concerns is also worthwhile for strengthening a supportive atmosphere.

Near-peer or peer coaching in medical education is often used by medical educators to enhance their own performance, but certainly has value for the medical students or trainees themselves. Peer coaching should be a mutually beneficial, nonevaluative relationship. It needs to be cooperative. In some settings the relationship is one-on-one and in others there are small groups. In a review of the literature most peer coaching is one-to-one and voluntary.[5] Self-assessment or reflection is a component of virtually all programs, and most coaching is goal-directed. Feedback is key, usually positive and constructive.

Peer coaching by learners at the same level of training (peers) or higher (near-peers) offers distinct advantages. Students and residents are often more receptive to feedback from individuals who have more contemporary learning

TABLE 5.1 Special Considerations for Group Coaching

Understand and balance shared and individual goals of students.
Establish safe space and a culture of curiosity and respect.
Assure engagement of all members.
Prepare for and mediate interpersonal conflicts.

Vignette 2

About 5 weeks into the first semester, Sam's formative course evaluations become available. Sam's coach, Dr. B, notices lackluster comments regarding Sam. He remembers her as a quiet student at orientation and decides to reach out to her. Sam, having forgotten about this valuable connection, is frustrated by the request to meet because she is overwhelmed and does not return the email. Because no relationship has been built to this point, Sam does not see the value of taking the time to meet with her coach.

As the semester continues, her grades start to reflect her despair. She starts to question why she was admitted to medical school. She reaches out to her family for help.

Thought Questions

1. How can Dr. B encourage Sam to reengage in their coaching relationship?
2. What questions could Dr. B ask to explore Sam's challenges?

experience and no formal evaluation role. For some coaching goals, the perspective of an individual who recently completed the same training may also provide highly valuable specifics compared with a coach whose training many years prior was significantly different.

Peer coaching can take many forms, but common features include a collaborative relationship free of competition, self-assessment, and goal-directed feedback.[6] Implementation of programs with these features requires the same commitment and responsibility as other forms of coaching but may be more challenging to achieve when both individuals are learners. Peer coaching in medicine benefits both the coach and coachee, and emphasizing this benefit to peer coaches may encourage mutual accountability.[7] Incorporation of coaching into curricular goals for students and residents is another method of assuring fuller investment by peer coaches.

ROLE OF THE COACH

The key to successful coaching lies in an understanding of the true role of the coach, and this role must be clear to both the coach and the student, resident, or group/team. As mentioned previously, although the coach may incorporate aspects of advising and mentoring, the focus here must be on the learner(s) and guiding them to self-reflection, ownership, and willingness to change. Thus all interactions are based on the intrinsic motivation of the learner. With this in mind, it is the coach who must insist on the learner setting the agenda and committing to the relationship. The coach provides the vehicle for the learner to reflect, set, and achieve goals and apply positive psychology tools. The coach does this through active listening, affirmation, asking good questions, and remaining available in a safe space to allow the learner to be open and honest without fear of judgment or evaluation. This process can be difficult—it is our nature to provide advice and to nurture. However, holding back, listening, affirming, and providing the learner the power to drive the relationship will help that learner toward building self-efficacy and professional identity as they become independent and confident. Positive psychology coaching has been shown to improve intern experience by using reflection, goal setting for success, and engaging in strengths exploration.[8] These tools may help build resilience and reduce emotional exhaustion. For more information on coaching models and frameworks, see Chapter 1.

The coaching program may offer faculty development, which is beneficial to coaches at all levels of experience. Time together with other coaches provides an opportunity to learn from each other through sharing. There may also be organized training sessions focused on the needs of the group. Often, workshops are designed to practice coaching skills. For example, role-playing is an effective activity that helps the coach become confident in their interactions with learners. The program should also provide the resources necessary should a situation develop in which a student or resident needs additional support outside the scope of the coach. The coach may refer learners to these other resources when appropriate and not feel that they need to have all of the answers. In fact, when a health or safety concern arises, it is imperative the learner be directed to appropriate professional assistance. Additional training, such as implicit bias training, wellness/stress reduction, mindfulness, curricular updates, and learning essentials, such as time management and study strategies, can increase the coach's toolbox in their approach to supporting student-identified needs while not crossing the boundaries of their role as defined by the institution's program.

Expectations and Boundaries

In the following sections of this chapter, we present suggested tools to assist coaches in creating effective relationships with their learners. Effective communication is a common theme of the best practices in this chapter. The coach is expected to be able to describe their role and their coaching program and reinforce the purpose of the relationship with the learner to add value to the time protected for meetings and activities. Learners must see the value of the relationship for progress to be made, otherwise they may see this as an infringement on their already-overcommitted time.

It is important for coaches to learn about the environment in which students and residents are immersed and to be familiar with competencies in relation to the developmental progress of a learner through each stage of training. Coaches should have a working knowledge of course/rotation structure and activities to enhance their ability to assist learners. However, with the proper access to resources coaches can be effective in their role without being content experts in the curriculum or advisers, thus building their credibility and relationship with their learners.

Coaching contracts can further open communication about expectations and boundaries for both the coach and the learner.

The Coaching Contract

A written agreement between the coach and the learner creates the foundation for understanding in the relationship, including both mutual responsibility and mutual understanding of where boundaries exist. Some suggested components of the contract include a brief statement describing the coaching program, a section that lists the responsibilities of both the learner and the coach, and space for mutual agreement of expectations and boundaries. The structure of the contract, the presence of a contract, and the process engaged can be very individualized by program. Although a coaching contract is a widely used tool, its effectiveness varies depending on buy-in and follow-through. A signature by both parties formalizes the agreement, and it is useful to refer back to the agreement regularly, especially if goals are included, thus forging the commitment.

Contracts may include a list of expectations, such as an agreement on confidentiality, regularity of meetings, open communication, how communication will occur (including boundaries such as late evening calls), acceptance of feedback, mutual respect considerations (such as being on time and responding in a timely manner), preparation for meetings, and setting the agenda for meetings. It is important to think of the contract as an opportunity to create the tone going forward and as a tool to assist in this important communication. We have included an example contract in Chapter 4 (Fig. 4.1), which may be expanded to include the number of goals appropriate for the learner and edited for different settings.

ORIENTATION TO COACHING

For both the learner and the coach, orientation to the coaching process is a critical first step. Coach orientation provides the overview and infrastructure necessary for consistency across the coaching program. Questions may range from the very basic and introductory to more specific, such as how to handle a crisis. For students and residents, the coaching program may be introduced in an informational session that highlights the goal of the coaching program. The role of coaching, as contrasted to mentoring or advising, should be outlined. Often, the program will provide a compendium of resources in the learning management system. Having a strong foundation and understanding will go a long way toward creating successful relationships.

Preparation

In advance of the first meeting, and all subsequent meetings, the coach should be aware of external pressures on their learners, such as curricular pressures, board exam timing, and upcoming transitions such as movement into clerkships or becoming a supervising resident. The coach should keep a record, even at a high level, to more easily move into a continuation of discussions or review of progress toward goals. These records include the coaching contract and goal-setting documents in addition to meeting notes that should be transparent to the learner. The learner must be prepared with an agenda and be open to discussion, bringing any challenges they currently face or anticipate. The coach may be required to review the learner's academic progress or contribute to the learner's use of feedback and appropriate responses. Additionally, the environment should be free from distraction, private, and safe.

The First Meeting

This first meeting sets the tone for future meetings and provides opportunity for the coach and student to begin the conversation about goal setting. This time should be used to open the door to communication, get to know each other, and begin building the trust that is so essential to a strong relationship. The contract may be developed at this meeting. This is also the time to introduce the idea of reflection, helping the learner identify their strengths and areas to improve. It is essential to now make the learner responsible for agenda setting for subsequent meetings.

Active listening is essential, and coaches should watch body language and ask open-ended questions. The coach should assure the learner is doing most of the talking and then summarize what they hear while providing empathy. Coaches should refrain from offering quick solutions, making assumptions, and being judgmental.

Tip: Do not allow too much time to pass before your second contact. Regular meetings initially set the ability to meet as needed down the road. Transitioning to "as needed" meetings too early will stall the goal of creating a trusting relationship.

Tip: Meet in person whenever possible, at least initially. Later, once the relationship is established, phone calls, virtual meetings, and emails may supplement in-person or online meetings.

THE SECOND AND SUBSEQUENT MEETINGS: ACTION PLANNING

As discussed at the first meeting, the learner should now create an agenda for ongoing meetings. It is important for students/trainees to feel ownership of their progress toward goals and a responsibility to the relationship. Some sessions may be designed by external pressures, such as regularly scheduled meetings in which the agenda and timing are driven by the program. Examples of this include time to review assessments, curricular progress, or transitions. However, the majority of the planning can remain with the learner, who decides what their personal goals are and how to get there. A reflection on well-being should be included. This is the opportunity to introduce the concept of the action plan and guide the learner toward success that is self-identified and thus intrinsically motivated. The learner may want the opportunity to meet with a coach to explore a specific issue, such as developing a plan toward a research project or to prepare for boards. Alternatively, the purpose may be much broader or long-range, such as becoming a successful resident. However, a generalized broad statement is much harder to recognize as achieved; coaches should assist learners toward envisioning specific aspects that define success.

Tips to guide the discussion:
- Use positive psychology coaching—discuss strengths and how to build on those strengths.
- Ask the learner what goals they have or what they would like to change.
- Ask the learner how they tackled a project in the past and why that strategy worked for them.
- Discuss the learner's comfort zone and how they might reach beyond their comfort to achieve their goal.
- Discuss persistence and strategies the learner used in the past.
- Discuss the master adaptive learner skills covered in Chapter 2.
- Introduce SMART goals: specific, measurable, achievable, relevant, and time-bound.
- Introduce WOOP goal setting: wish, outcome, obstacle, and plan.

Action Planning

As part of the goal setting with the learner, another useful tool is an action plan. A formal action plan can be developed as an activity with the learner by encouraging the learner to brainstorm short- and long-term goals. Jotting down ideas to build the action plan together and then giving the learner "homework" for further reflection may contribute to relationship building and trust. The learner can either use a worksheet designed to walk them through the process or may design their own plan by including steps necessary to reach their specific goal, a timeline for each step, and how each step will be measured. The learner should identify their ultimate goal and be able to identify how they will know they are successful in meeting the short-term steps toward their goal. Learners should think about the resources that will be required and potential barriers to overcome. As a coach, one guides the learner through this planning and helps the learner see their mini milestones, reinforcing the good work accomplished together, followed by celebration of success. Goal-setting frameworks such as WOOP and SMART tools are discussed in the next section.

Self-assessment by learners is central to all coaching programs and may be guided by reflection exercises or other techniques such as motivational advising. This approach uses motivational interview questions, typically open-ended, to coach the learner toward making an internally motivated commitment to a behavioral change and/or professional challenge. The coach guides coachees to counteract ambivalence to change and adopt positive behavioral changes.[7] Reflection exercises use either open-ended guiding questions or a series of Likert-scaled questions regarding values, attitudes, and behaviors. Providing dedicated time for both completion and coaching around these exercises can greatly improve their utility.

Goal-Setting Strategies

There are a number of strategies a coach can use to help the learner through the planning process. Central among these various approaches is the idea that each goal must be achievable and measurable, which helps to secure the motivation toward improvement.

SMART: Specific, Measurable, Achievable, Relevant, and Time-bound

This type of goal setting walks the learner through their action plan. First, make the goal specific, focused, and not too broad. The goal should be measurable and achievable in order to maintain motivation and improve chances of reaching the goal. The "R" can be relevant or realistic. The coach can ask appropriate questions of the learner to help focus the goal to being within reach. And finally, time creates impetus and urgency. Think of deadlines as motivators toward success.[9]

WOOP Goal Setting: Wish, Outcome, Obstacle, and Plan

This form of goal setting seems to be uniquely suited for individuals in a coaching program, as it provides imaginary exercises that increase goal commitment and behavioral change compared with other methods. The wish is something that is important to the learner, such as "I want to be a better team member in my anatomy group." The outcome is the learner's single best outcome, "I want to improve communication with my peers." The obstacle should be something internal, such as overcoming shyness or feelings of anxiety when speaking in front of others. Finally, the plan should be a specific action taken when the obstacle arises. For example, at the next team meeting, the learner plans to purposefully speak up and provide a prepared fact to help in the next dissection. WOOP goal setting has been implemented and studied in medical education, resulting in an increased goal-directed study within anesthesiology residents.[10]

INSTITUTION-SPECIFIC GOALS

Medical schools and residency programs may use coaching for achieving a variety of institution-specific goals (Table 5.2). A common theme of many programs is maintaining a stable, long-term relationship between a faculty coach and the learner through the duration of training. Such continuity positions coaches to follow the academic progress of their students and residents and assist with identification of and early intervention for deficiencies.[11] Coach-mediated academic monitoring can be particularly beneficial when coupled with performance dashboards and well-coordinated remediation systems.[12] Similarly, coaching programs in medical schools are often integrated with clinical skills curricula to have the same faculty coaches teaching physical examination and clinical reasoning.[13] Maintaining educational continuity can improve standardization of teaching clinical skills and enable systems of competency-based academic progression. Other programs

TABLE 5.2   School-Specific Goals for Coaching Programs
Follow academic progress and facilitate early intervention for deficiencies.
Monitor and assist clinical skills development.
Review learner's ability to provide and receive evaluation feedback.
Foster professional identity formation.
Facilitate career planning.
Use student-driven individual learning plans.
Implement well-being curriculum.

may focus on professional development, including the ability to provide effective feedback and accept feedback from others.

Professional development includes professional identity formation, which is a continuous process that begins even prior to matriculation into medical school. Early deliberate coaching of professional identity formation can positively affect learners' acquisition of higher levels of professional identity.[14] Furthermore, longitudinal coaching facilitates career planning. Through formation of close relationships, faculty coaches develop a holistic understanding of learners' goals and can better assist their navigation of career choices. Likewise, long-term coaching relationships can empower students and residents to use individual learning plans. Using appreciative inquiry, coaches can guide learners to self-identify personal and professional goals that are realistic and consistent with their values.[15] Coaching programs also provide a reliable format to assure accountability and follow-through, which are key to the success of individual learning plans.[16]

With recognition of the increasing problem of physician distress and burnout, many medical schools and residency programs have implemented curricula focused on improving well-being. The majority of drivers of learner unwellness are organizational in nature, but there is evidence for benefit of individual interventions, including mindfulness exercises, meditation, yoga, and self-care workshops.[17,18] Other well-being activities heavily emphasize community building and mattering. Although developing interpersonal relationships between learners and strengthening learners' sense of meaning and purpose do not require the involvement of a faculty coach, coaches can improve achievement of these elements. Coaches can facilitate the sometimes challenging initiation of community building between individuals of varying beliefs and backgrounds. Faculty coaches also reinforce learners' sense of purpose and belonging by engaging with them as members of a shared professional community.

Tips for Group Sessions

Establishment of a safe space in which all individuals mutually respect each other is absolutely necessary for successful group coaching.[19] Coaches must establish this culture at the beginning of a group's formation. Although stating behavior standards or having learners and coaches sign a letter of agreement may be beneficial, having a group develop its own charter with expectations and goals can be more impactful. Collaborative creation of a set of responsibilities regarding one another sets the group on a stronger foundation of mutual accountability than does agreement to external rules. Self-derived covenants also instill greater investment in the coaching program from group members.

As with any meeting, the leader must assure engagement of all members. Less extroverted individuals may be hesitant to engage in discussions, particularly when others are outspoken or the subject matter is sensitive. Starting with "icebreaker questions" can help draw in learners. Examples include having everyone tell the group their favorite free-time activity and sharing what they are thankful for. Faculty coaches should use open-ended questions and preface them with statements to assure the group that members may have differing opinions but all opinions matter. When disagreements occur, the coach must be ready to tactfully address rather than avoid the subject. In some circumstances, disputes and personality differences between group members (including the coach and a learner) may be so substantial that they disrupt the dynamics of the entire group. Separately engaging with the individuals in conflict may allow for easing of tensions and resetting of relationships. Because learning to work with individuals with different beliefs and personalities is a key part of becoming a physician, only in rare circumstances should group assignments be changed.

Confidentiality

Establishing a trusting individual or peer-coaching relationship is vital. Confidentiality must be strictly maintained, and a signed coaching agreement between participants should be considered. Coaching programs must also ensure that faculty are never in evaluation roles for their coachees and that peer coaching activities encourage collaboration and not competition.

Incorporating Feedback

Feedback is an integral part of medical training, but it has a unique context within a coaching program. As a coach, one's primary role is to guide a learner through self-exploration of feedback that they have received from other sources rather than directly provide feedback. The coach may also provide valuable guidance to learners as they themselves must learn to provide feedback to peers, junior learners, and faculty. Within a coaching relationship there are instances when both coach and learner must provide and receive feedback (e.g., learner providing feedback on coaching efficacy or coach providing feedback to learner on their interactions with peers during group sessions). Coaches may also be placed in a role where they are using coaching techniques mixed with feedback, if they are directly observing a performance/skill. Furthermore, coaches must understand optimal feedback methods to encourage learners to effectively seek and assimilate feedback that can be used in coaching sessions. Learners are often extremely desirous of feedback yet may fail to actively seek it because of fear of criticism.

TABLE 5.3   **Features of Effective Feedback**
Goal-directed: targeted to outcomes the student values
Actionable: specific recommendations that are appropriate for skill level
Timely: communicated as soon as possible after performance/behavior is encountered
Continuous: incorporating follow-up of previous feedback and interventions taken
Consistent with established expectations

Based on Wiggins, G. Seven keys to effective feedback. *Educational Leadership.* 2012;70(1):10–16.

TABLE 5.4   **Characteristics of Effective Feedback-Seeking Behavior**
Confirm performance expectations at start of educational relationship.
Solicit feedback frequently (e.g., at end of each clinic with preceptor, at end of a week on an inpatient rotation).
Include self-assessment of areas for improvement that a student or supervisor has identified.
Seek feedback in a private setting that allows for candid discussion.

Provision of quality feedback includes several key elements (Table 5.3). Feedback should be goal focused and, as much as possible, tied directly to learner self-assessment.[20] Learners are generally more open to feedback on targets identified through self-evaluation, and the impact of coaching on these topics will be higher yield because they are directed at the learner's specific areas of concern. However, it is important to assure that both self-assessments and feedback are aligned with curricular goals and expectations. Feedback should also be part of a continuous improvement process and provided frequently in a timely fashion. When learners develop plans for improvement, a coach should set expectations for following up with the learner at a set point in time.

Seeking and assimilating feedback is also a skill many learners struggle with and can improve upon with coaching. As with feedback provision, expectations should be set by coaches that students will solicit feedback in all relevant educational settings. Coaches should reinforce the characteristics of effective feedback-seeking behavior (Table 5.4). It is also helpful to call out and discourage several mistakes in seeking feedback, including: avoidance due to concern that a supervisor is too busy; timing solicitation to occur after positive experiences only; and pursuing feedback only from supervisors a learner personally likes.[21]

Coaches should guide students on appropriate processing of feedback. One approach to coaching around feedback is the R2C2 model developed by Sargeant and colleagues in 2015. The model uses four phases: (1) build rapport and relationship, (2) explore reactions to the feedback, (3) explore understanding of the content, and (4) coach for performance change.[22] All these steps are congruent with general coaching concepts that emphasize developing a trusting, collaborative relationship with a learner and guiding them to self-analyze and develop their own improvement plans.

Receiving criticism of one's performance can be difficult, and learners must be coached to retain an open mind and remain committed to improvement. Feedback should not be taken personally; instead, it should be accepted without argument as a valid perception of their performance. When feedback is factually incorrect or incongruent with previous expectations, the receiver should seek clarification of goals and objectives. If receiving only positive or vague feedback, learners should share their self-identified areas for improvement and ask for suggestions. Finally, after receiving feedback, learners should develop with the supervisor a plan for improvement and follow up and share this plan with their coach.

Record Keeping

Documentation of meetings can serve several purposes: proof of mandatory meetings, longitudinal tracking of goals, and reminder of previous discussions. However, it is imperative that coaches adhere to institutional requirements and federal regulations. The Family Educational Rights and Privacy Act (FERPA) ensures that students over age 18 years have the right to review all information within their educational files.[23] Coaches should keep this in mind with all documentation but also not allow it to serve as a deterrent from recording important information from their discussions. By maintaining transparency of record keeping, coaches can provide a useful record of coaching sessions and reinforce the importance of the feedback process. Keeping records that are not available to the learner presents important pitfalls. First, such information is never totally inaccessible to students at public institutions because it is subject to Freedom of Information requests. Second, maintaining such records in a nonsecure location could result in a violation of FERPA if the information was accessed by others without the student's permission. Most importantly, privately documenting learner information undermines trust and contradicts the growth mindset approach to feedback upon which coaching is based.

CLOSING THE RELATIONSHIP

All coaching partnerships eventually end. For programs that pair the same coach and learner for the duration of medical school or residency, this conclusion occurs with graduation. In other programs, coaching only occurs for part of a student's medical education, and the coaching relationship closes with that period's completion. With these successful transitions, coaches and learners should celebrate achievements, reflect on their journey, and discuss future goals. In addition to reinforcing key areas to continue focusing improvement efforts, coaches should consider offering their ongoing advice and support.

In some circumstances, a coach may unexpectedly leave a coaching program (e.g., due to departure from the institution). When such an event occurs, a coach should provide closure with the learner by meeting to discuss their progress thus far and targets for continued focus. The coach should also seek the learner's permission to discuss their coaching experience with the coach's replacement to assure a smooth transition. If a learner leaves a coaching program, the coach should conduct an exit interview with the learner to show their support and determine how they may be able to assist the learner outside of the coaching partnership.

Rarely, irreconcilable differences may develop between a coach and coachee that necessitate dissolving the relationship. Before reaching this point, every attempt should be made to salvage the relationship. In most cases, one-on-one discussions that revisit the goals of coaching and acknowledging personal differences will be sufficient to continue the collaboration. When necessary, a mediator, such as the coaching program coordinator, can also engage in these discussions. Only when all reasonable efforts have failed should the coaching partnership be formally ended.

Vignette 3

The plight of Sam could have been avoided if better communication plans were in place. The coach, who doesn't realize Sam is struggling, does not react until failing grades begin to appear. Sam, feeling all alone, does not reach out to someone who can provide a different perspective and help focus on strategies for well-being. Earlier, regular meetings to create the relationship and trust would have allowed for action planning toward a number of attainable goals: balance for wellness; study strategies that may include study partners, time management, and review skills; and perhaps a personal goal to create friendships with other students who can form a support network.

Thought Questions

1. What can Dr. B do now to improve Sam's experience as a first-year medical student?
2. Imagine Sam is an intern rather than a medical student. How is the transition to residency similar to the transition to medical school? How can coaching improve her experience under these circumstances?
3. What other scenarios can you think of where coaching can be inserted to improve student well-being?
4. When is it appropriate to enlist the help of other resources at the school?

TAKE-HOME POINTS

Effective communication strategies for both the coach and the learner include:

1. Structure: A good coaching program will have the infrastructure to support both coach and learner. The structure can be as simple as preset dates for meetings, preset activities to engage, and/or group meetings to encourage relationship building. The meetings should take place in relaxed, safe spaces.
2. Focus: There should be intentional effort to direct questions back to the learner to keep the focus on self-discovery in a respectful and nonthreatening manner.
3. Discovery: The coach should ask open-ended questions as discussed earlier in this chapter.
4. Contract: This involves agreement between the coach and coachee, including program goals and scope of the relationship, as well as boundaries and expectations.
5. Goal setting: Self-reflection and communication between the learner and coach will contribute toward regular review of goals and move the learner toward self-improvement.
6. Frequency: Start the relationship with planned, short-range, time-framed meetings and agree on the frequency of meetings in the coaching contract. This item can be revisited as the relationship develops.

QUESTIONS FOR FURTHER THOUGHT

1. Consider the culture and needs of your setting. Which of the coaching program types best fits your needs? Focus groups may help you decide on one or a combination of coaching types.
2. How can faculty development programming best support your coaching program?
3. Does your program provide adequate support resources to your coaches? How can you improve this support?
4. Checking in is important both for coaches and coachees. If you are a coach, are you checking in regularly with your coachees? If you are a coaching director, are you checking in with your coaches?
5. Consider opportunities for improved feedback. Think of how you may use the feedback loop to improve communication, both between you and your coachees, as well as coaching for better feedback.

ANNOTATED BIBLIOGRAPHY

Hauer KE, Iverson N, Quach A, Yuan P, Kaner S, Boscardin C, Fostering medical students' lifelong learning skills with a dashboard, coaching and learning planning. *Perspect Med Educ.* 2018;7:311–31.
Describes and analyzes implementation of a successful, comprehensive coaching program at a top-tier medical school. Lead author is a recognized expert in medical education coaching.

Lovell B. What do we know about coaching in medical education? A literature review. *Med Educ.* 2018;52(4): 376–390.
A literature review of 21 papers focusing on coaching interventions in three categories: well-being and resilience; improved nontechnical skills; and improved technical skills. The review concludes that the strongest evidence of coaching effectiveness is in teaching of technical skills. Paper calls for further studies investigating coaching in medical students and doctors.

Reynolds AK. Academic coaching for learners in medical education: Twelve tips for the learning specialist. *Med Teach.* 2020;42(6):616–621.
Concise summary of key components of coaching in medical education. Provides practical advice for individuals engaged as academic coaches.

Sargeant J, Lockyer J, Mann K, et al. Facilitated reflective performance feedback: developing an evidence- and theory-based model that builds relationship, explores reactions and content, and coaches for performance change (R2C2). *Acad Med.* 2015; 90(12):1698–1706.
Outlines the development and performance of a coaching model that is widely cited and used within undergraduate and graduate medical education.

REFERENCES

1. Lovell B. What do we know about coaching in medical education? A literature review. *Med Educ.* 2018;52(4):376–390.
2. Petty GM, Lingham T. Coaching teamwork in the classroom using an innovative team-coaching process. *Nurs Educ Perspect.* 2019;40(2):118–120.
3. Manger T, Thatcher C. A synergy between peer evaluation and student coaching in team-based learning: coach review of peer evaluations improves student acceptance. *Med Sci Educ.* 2020;30:597–600.
4. Malling B, de Lasson L, Just E, Stegeager N. How group coaching contributes to organisational understanding among newly graduated doctors. *BMC Med Educ.* 2020;20:193.
5. Schwellnus H, Carnahan H. Peer-coaching with health care professionals: What is the current status of the literature and what are the key components necessary in peer-coaching? A scoping review. *Med Teach.* 2014;36(1):38–46.
6. Yu TC, Wilson NC, Singh PP, et al. Medical students-as-teachers: a systematic review of peer-assisted teaching during medical school. *Adv Med Educ Pract.* 2011;2:157–172.
7. Parekh K, Benningfield M, Burrows H, et al. Motivational advising workshop: utilizing motivational interviewing theory to facilitate and engage intrinsic motivation to change learners' behavior. *Med Ed PORTAL.* 2018;14:10751.
8. Palamara K, Kauffman C, Chang Y, et al. Professional development coaching for residents: results of a 3-year positive psychology coaching intervention. *J Gen Intern Med.* 2018;33:1842–1844.
9. Lawlor K, Hornyak M. Smart goals: how the application of smart goals can contribute to the achievement of student learning outcomes. *Developments in Business Simulation and Experiential Learning.* 2012:39.
10. Saddawi-Konefka D, Baker K, Guarino A, et al. changing resident physician studying behaviors: a randomized, comparative effectiveness trial of goal setting versus use of WOOP. *J Grad Med Educ.* 2017;9(4):451–457.
11. Osterberg LG, Goldstein E, Hatem DS, et al. Back to the future: what learning communities offer to medical education. *J Med Educ Curric Dev.* January 2016.
12. Hauer KE, Iverson N, Quach A, Yuan P, Kaner S, Boscardin C. Fostering medical students' lifelong learning skills with a dashboard, coaching and learning planning. *Perspect Med Educ.* 2018;7:311–331.
13. Jackson MB, Keen M, Wenrich MD, et al. Impact of a pre-clinical clinical skills curriculum on student performance in third-year clerkships. *J Gen Intern Med.* 2009;24(8):929–933.
14. Cruess SR, Cruess RL, Steinert Y. Supporting the development of a professional identity: General principles. *Med Teach.* 2019;41(6):641–649.

15. Sandars J, Murdoch-Eaton D. Appreciative inquiry in medical education. *Med Teach*. 2017;39(2):123–127.

16. Challis M. AMEE Medical Education Guide No. 19: Personal learning plans. *Med Teach*.200;22(3):225–236.

17. West CP, Dyrbye LN, Erwin PJ, Shanafelt TD. Interventions to prevent and reduce physician burnout: a systematic review and meta-analysis. *Lancet*. 2016;388(10057):2272–2281.

18. Zhang XJ, Song Y, Jiang T, et al. Interventions to reduce burnout of physicians and nurses. *Medicine (Baltimore)*. 2020;99(26):e20992.

19. Reynolds AK. Academic coaching for learners in medical education: Twelve tips for the learning specialist. *Med Teach*. 2020;42(6):616–621.

20. Wiggins G. Seven keys to effective feedback. *Educational Leadership*. 2012;70(1):10–16.

21. Crommelinck M, Anseel F. Understanding and encouraging feedback-seeking behaviour: a literature review. *Med Educ*. 2013;47:232–241.

22. Sargeant J, Lockyer J, Mann K, et al. Facilitated reflective performance feedback: developing an evidence- and theory-based model that builds relationship, explores reactions and content, and coaches for performance change (R2C2). *Acad Med*. 2015;90(12):1698–1706.

23. Family Educational Rights and Privacy Act (FERPA), US Department of Education. https://www2.ed.gov/policy/gen/guid/fpco/ferpa/index.html. Accessed July 26, 2021.

Applications of Coaching

Ronda Mourad, Archana Pradhan, and Amy Miller Juve

LEARNING OBJECTIVES

1. Discuss developmental principles that are foundational to all potential applications of coaching.
2. Describe how coaching can be used in eight applications across the medical education continuum

of learning—for the development of a master adaptive learner.

3. Highlight specific coaching tools and competencies that are key success factors for coaching applications.

CHAPTER OUTLINE

CHAPTER SUMMARY

Based on the principles and frameworks of several scientific domains (e.g., positive psychology, behavioral psychology, motivational interviewing, motivation, adult learning, adult development, and mindfulness), coaching empowers the coachee to adopt a proactive approach to visioning future self, goal setting, optimizing growth, and expanding potential (Chapter 3). By leveraging their strengths and learning to create visions (imagining ideal outcomes or future self) and goals (stepping-stones to get there) that are intrinsically motivated, coachees gain competence in setting a direction for development. Over time, coachees develop a sense of mastery in overcoming challenges and obstacles using strengths and resources. All of this helps bring about self-directed learning, positive change, and growth.

Coaching can be useful to learners across the continuum of training and ideally continues throughout their careers as independent practitioners. With practice, individuals can master skills required to coach others, and ultimately, to coach themselves through any personal or professional challenge across many different settings.

INTRODUCTION

Coaching is designed to help guide learners of all stages move from where they are to where they want to be in a manner driven by themselves. The process encourages learners to create intrinsically motivated goals linked to their strengths, core values, and long-term vision. Although the strongest evidence for coaching in medical education focuses on technical skills, we can use existing coaching modalities to coach learners through the process of choosing a specialty, identifying research mentors, developing leadership skills, adapting to change, embracing new technical challenges, or committing to personal health and wellness.[1] The most effective coaching relationships provide opportunities for learners to self-reflect and explore possibilities in a confidential space free of evaluation and judgment.

This chapter focuses on applications of coaching specific to development of a master adaptive learner in the medical sciences. The terms *coachee* and *learner* are used interchangeably and can be applied to learners at all stages of their careers, including faculty who are committed to a profession where lifelong learning and continual process improvement is expected.

Coaching can be applied to maximize potential and growth for learners across many venues and at all stages of their careers, during training and beyond, when we follow the core principles and frameworks of coaching (Fig. 6.1).

PROFESSIONAL IDENTITY FORMATION AND CAREER DEVELOPMENT

Professional identity formation is an evolving, lifelong process in which an individual internalizes the core values, beliefs, and actions of a profession.[2,3] Navigating and reflecting upon a variety of experiences throughout the course of development, whether that be a medical student developing their identity as a physician or a faculty member developing their identity as an educator, helps an individual form their professional identity.

Coaching serves as a catalyst to help a learner make meaning of and learn from their failures and successes, their surrounding environment, and their interactions with others as they work to internalize their developing professional identity. Using prompts from the professional identity essay (PIE) is one way a coach can engage learners to support the development of and potentially assess their coachee's professional identity formation (Table 6.1).[4]

For example, in the vignette, our third-year medical student, Joe, witnesses an interaction between his preceptor and a patient that puzzles him. The preceptor is 20 minutes late to a patient's scheduled appointment start time. The preceptor rushes into the room without apologizing or explaining why he is late. The appointment is short and hurried, and Joe perceives that the patient left the appointment frustrated and with unanswered questions. Joe is hesitant to discuss his concerns directly with his preceptor because of the inherent hierarchy in their relationship, but speaking with his coach, who ideally is removed from an evaluative role, allows Joe to explore his ideas in a confidential and judgment-free space without fear of potential retribution or affecting the relationship with his preceptor.

As Joe talks to his coach about his observations, the coach can guide him through questions from the PIE to help him identify environmental factors, professional responsibilities, and patient expectations that may have

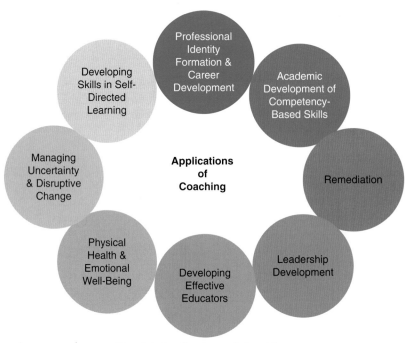

Fig. 6.1 Applications of Coaching.

TABLE 6.1 Prompting Questions from the Professional Identity Essay (PIE)
What does being a member of the medical profession mean to you? How did you come to this understanding?
What do you expect of yourself as you work toward becoming a full-fledged physician?
What will the profession expect of you?
What conflicts do you experience or expect to experience between your responsibility to yourself and others—patients, family, and profession? How do you resolve them?
What would be the worst consequence for you if you failed to live up to the expectations you have set for yourself?
What would be the worst consequence for you if you failed to live up to the expectations of your patients?
What would be the worst consequence for you if you failed to live up to what society expects of physicians? How did you come to this understanding?
Think of a physician you consider an exemplar of professionalism. Describe why you chose this person, illustrating with an incident or pattern of decisions or actions that supports your choice.
Reflect on your experiences in medical school or in the community that have been critical in fostering change in your understanding of what it means to be a professional—to be a physician.

Modified for use in medicine. From Kalet A, Buckvar-Keltz L, Harnik V, et al. Measuring professional identity formation early in medical school. *Med Teach.* 2017;39(3):255–261.

Vignette

Joe is a third-year medical student who is struggling with professionalism during his general surgery core clerkship. He is consistently late to didactic sessions, requires frequent reminders to complete assignments, and is disrespectful toward hospital staff. He has received a below-average score for the core competency of professionalism on his recent evaluation. When his clerkship director meets with him to review his performance, she informs him that he will be required to meet with a coach equipped to assist with remediation of professionalism. Joe is unconcerned about the below-average professionalism score, stating that he is exceeding expectations in medical knowledge and that most of his patients have expressed positive feedback about his bedside manner.

Thought Questions

1. How can coaches and coachees approach remediation with a growth mindset that removes stigma, maximizes growth, and empowers learners to transcend their own challenges?
2. How can coaches foster self-directed learning and self-motivation in learners who are mandated to engage in coaching as part of a remediation plan?
3. How can coaching help the learner explore the ways their actions are perceived by others and potentially affecting patient encounters?

contributed to the preceptor's actions. The coach can then help Joe explore his intrinsic motivators, values, and beliefs in relation to how he would approach that same patient encounter if he were the preceptor.

Each experience, especially if challenging, is an opportunity for the coach to provide a safe space for the learner to understand the tensions they feel in relation to how they will practice when they enter the profession. At times, helping the learner navigate the tensions they feel may require the coach to guide the learner toward additional resources, such as a mentor. Maintaining this distinction between coach and mentor preserves the "learner as expert" role during coaching sessions, so that over time, learners better develop a sense of mastery and self-efficacy in imagining an ideal outcome, solving problems, and resolving conflicts, while still allowing them additional opportunities outside of coaching to seek external expertise from a mentor when necessary.

ACADEMIC DEVELOPMENT OF COMPETENCY-BASED SKILLS

An academic coach is a person assigned to facilitate learners achieving their fullest potential.[5] Coaching for academic development in the context of medical education often focuses on teaching learners to use deliberate practice strategies to achieve a level of competency in any or all of the established Accreditation Council for Graduate Medical

Education (ACGME) core areas: medical knowledge, patient care, interpersonal and communication skills, professionalism, systems-based practice, and practice-based learning and improvement. Coaches may work with coachees to develop plans to practice repetitive and structured activities that focus on cognitive skill development through rigorous assessments and specific feedback.[6]

For example, academic coaches can work with students who are preparing for United States Medical Licensing Exam (USMLE) Step 1. These coaches can help students identify specific medical knowledge deficits by reviewing learners' objective assessments and performance data. As these assessments are reviewed, it is important coaches create opportunities for learner self-assessment. Explaining an evidenced-based framework such as Bloom's taxonomy to the learner and following up with questions, such as "What levels best describe your study strategies for this test?" may help the learner with self-assessment.[7] Inquiring about prior successes, such as "What strategies helped you prepare for the MCAT?" can also assist the learner in creating new goals based on leveraging their strengths.

Beyond the needs assessment, coaches can help learners create individualized learning plans to overcome medical knowledge deficiencies through strength-based appreciative inquiry and developing specific, measurable, achievable, relevant, and time-based (SMART) goals (Chapter 3). With consistent practice, leveraging their strengths to create and ultimately to achieve realistic goals fosters confidence and, over time, a sense of mastery and self-efficacy as they recognize all the successes that are possible.[8]

These same principles can be used to help a coachee with academic development in other arenas such as performance coaching in clinical skills development, clinical reasoning, psychomotor skill acquisition, or research skills development like performing a thorough literature search or graphically presenting findings (Chapter 7).

REMEDIATION OF SPECIFIC COMPETENCIES: REFRAMING THE APPROACH TO REMEDIATION

Coaching allows faculty and learners to reframe remediation into a process that is proactive, learner driven, and strengths based. Although coaching is applicable to remediating any core competency, an approach to remediating professionalism is discussed in this section. Addressing unprofessional behaviors in a judgment-free space can be particularly challenging for both parties. When individuals demonstrate behaviors that are perceived as unprofessional, assumptions may be made about their personal character, attitudes, or values.[9]

These assumptions may lead to an oversimplified or punitive intervention that can then create shame or defensive reactions that hinder growth and remediation. Educators can reframe professionalism remediation by challenging such assumptions. This includes recognizing that individuals with professional core values can demonstrate unprofessional behaviors at times, guiding learners to identify environmental factors that contribute to their actions, exploring strengths and resources learners can use to correct their attitudes and behaviors, implementing a pedagogical response using targeted coaching, and acknowledging that this process is complex and dynamic over time.[9]

Through self-reflection tools and strength-based appreciative inquiry (Chapter 3), coaches can help learners recognize discrepancies between their intentions and their behaviors (or perceived behaviors) in order to reconcile how their actions affect others. One useful reflection tool is Peterson and Seligman's Values in Action Inventory of Strengths (VIA-IS). A modified version of the VIA (Table 6.2) was developed for use at the Internal Medicine Residency's Professional Coaching Program at the Massachusetts General Hospital,[10] which, through reflection and self-discovery, can help coachees link their values and strengths to their professional aspirations and long-term vision.

A suggested framework for remediation is to pose open questions on professional identity development to stimulate discussions about professionalism (Table 6.3).[11] Minimizing shame or stigma and displaying empathy, particularly when coaching, are essential. Encouraging coachees to create goals that are linked to their core values, aspirations, and intrinsic motivators (rather than focusing solely on externally mandated or punitive goals) is paramount to achieving authentic, sustainable change. Furthermore, helping learners design goals in this way can inspire them to strive to surpass minimum requirements, maximize their growth potential, and eventually master a designated competency.

LEADERSHIP DEVELOPMENT

Coaching to develop leadership skills in all learners in the medical education continuum is critical to improving patient and health care organization outcomes, although coaching models for leadership development in medical education are sparse.[12] However, the tenets that the American Medical Association (AMA) Accelerating Change in Medical Education Consortium has established as key to a medical school leadership curriculum mirror coaching principles: (1) leadership starts with understanding oneself and one's leadership values, (2) leadership is about inspiring and leading change, and (3) leadership is about guiding teams and fostering accountability to one

TABLE 6.2	**Peterson and Seligman's Values in Action Inventory of Strengths**
	FOR EACH STRENGTH circle how much this is "like you" 1 = not like me, 10% or less; 5 = like me, nearly 100% of the time
HEAD	**Wisdom and Knowledge**
Creativity 1 2 3 4 5	Trying new ways of approaching medical problems is crucial to who you are. Although you are not averse to conventional methods, you enjoy exploring alternative and innovative perspectives. You are never content with doing something the conventional way if a more effective way is possible.
Curiosity 1 2 3 4 5	You are curious about your patients and their problems. You are always asking questions and find many subjects and topics fascinating. You love exploration and discovery, even without an immediate practical application.
Love of learning 1 2 3 4 5	You love learning new things and teaching them to others. You get excited by new medical knowledge that you can incorporate and teach to others. Professionally and in general, you gain pleasure by learning and teaching on a wide array of topics.
Open mindedness 1 2 3 4 5	Thinking things through and examining them from different perspectives are important aspects of who you are. You do not jump to clinical conclusions, and you consider others' input when making decisions. You are able to change your mind when judgment indicates it.
Perspective 1 2 3 4 5	Although you may not consider yourself wise, your colleagues hold this view of you. They value your perspective on cases and professional challenges and turn to you for advice. You have a way of looking at the world that makes sense to others and to yourself.
HEART	**Strengths of Humanity**
Kindness 1 2 3 4 5	You enjoy doing good deeds for others and are altruistic. You tend to be selfless and enjoy community service. You find helping a patient or colleague deeply satisfying.
Capacity to love and be loved 1 2 3 4 5	You value close relations with patients and colleagues, particularly those in which caring is reciprocated. The people you feel most close to are the same people who feel closest to you.
Social intelligence 1 2 3 4 5	You are tuned into the feelings of your patients, families, and coworkers. You know how to fit into different social situations, and how to put others at ease. You bring calm to challenging clinical encounters.
COURAGE	
Authenticity 1 2 3 4 5	You are an honest person, not only by speaking the truth but by living and working in a genuine and authentic way. You are down to earth and without pretense; you are a "real" person. In clinical situations you err on the side of full disclosure.
Bravery 1 2 3 4 5	You are a courageous person who does not shrink from threat, challenge, difficulty, or pain. You are not someone who avoids challenging cases. You speak up for what is right even if there is opposition. You act on your convictions and bounce back from failures.
Persistence 1 2 3 4 5	You work hard to finish what you start, regardless of obstacles. No matter the project, you "check the boxes" in timely fashion. You do not get distracted when you work, you take responsibility for and learn from errors, and you take satisfaction in completing tasks.
Zest 1 2 3 4 5	Regardless of what you do, you approach it with excitement and energy. You don't do your job halfheartedly. Your career and every clinical encounter carries an aspect of adventure for you. You tend to energize others.

Continued

TABLE 6.2	Peterson and Seligman's Values in Action Inventory of Strengths—cont'd
COMMUNITY	**Strengths of Justice**
Fairness 1 2 3 4 5	Treating patients and coworkers fairly is one of your abiding principles. You are nonhierarchical in your approach, give everyone a chance, and do not let your personal feelings bias your decisions about people.
Leadership 1 2 3 4 5	You excel at leadership, including motivating patients to work toward health goals, fostering effective relationships, and managing conflict in your team to work toward a common vision. You preserve harmony within the team by making everyone feel included. You do a good job organizing activities and seeing that they happen.
Teamwork 1 2 3 4 5	You identify well as a member of a team. You are a loyal and dedicated teammate. You always do your share and are motivated by a sense of common purpose. You work hard for the success of team.
TEMPERANCE	
Forgiveness/mercy 1 2 3 4 5	You are empathetic and forgive those who you believe have done you wrong. You give challenging patients and colleagues a second chance and move beyond past conflicts. Your guiding principle is mercy and not revenge. You are fueled by empathy and perspective, not guilt or fear.
Modesty/humility 1 2 3 4 5	You do not seek the spotlight, preferring to let your accomplishments speak for themselves. You do not regard yourself as special. You are not condescending, and others recognize and value your modesty.
Prudence 1 2 3 4 5	You are a careful and conscientious physician, and your choices are consistently prudent and strategic ones, oriented toward a long-term vision. You do not say or do things that you might later regret.
Self-regulation, self-control 1 2 3 4 5	You self-consciously regulate what you feel and what you do, so you stay in a state of self-control. You are a disciplined, nonimpulsive person. You are in control of your appetites and emotions.
TRANSCENDENCE	
Appreciation of beauty and excellence 1 2 3 4 5	You notice and appreciate beauty, excellence, and/or skilled performance in all domains of life and work, from enhancing function to nature to art to science to everyday patient care.
Gratitude 1 2 3 4 5	You are aware of the good things that happen to you, and you don't take them for granted. You try to take the time to express your gratitude to everyone from medical students to nurses.
Hope 1 2 3 4 5	You expect the best in the future, and you work to achieve it. You believe that the future is something on which you can have an impact. Your belief in positive outcomes helps you see possibilities and new plans of action where others may not.
Humor 1 2 3 4 5	You use humor comfortably with patients. Bringing smiles to other people is important to you. You are able to see the light side of all situations and do so to defuse negative situations.
Religiousness and spirituality 1 2 3 4 5	You have strong and coherent beliefs about the purpose and meaning of the universe. You know where you and your work fit into the larger scheme, providing a reservoir of calm and a buffer from stress. Your beliefs shape your actions and are a source of comfort to you.

This modified version of Peterson and Seligman's Values in Action Inventory of Strengths is used in the internal medicine residency's professional coaching program at Massachusetts General Hospital. Modified from Palamara K, Kauffman C, Stone VE, Barzi H, Donelan K. Promoting success: A professional development coaching program for interns in medicine. *J Grad Med Educ*. 2015;7(4):630–637.

TABLE 6.3   Using Open Questions on Professional Identity to Stimulate Discussions about Professionalism

What professional goals do you want to accomplish during your medical career?

What personal goals do you want to achieve during your medical career?

What ideal physician characteristics drew you to pursue a career in medicine? Which of these attributes or values do you already emulate? Which ones are you still working toward achieving?

What factors that *you control* in your professional life can help you achieve these goals? What strengths can you leverage to get you there? What factors that *you control* could prevent you from achieving these goals?

How do persistent unprofessional behaviors affect patient care or other professional outcomes?

Adapted from Iserson KV. Talking about professionalism through the lens of professional identity. *AEM Educ Train.* 2018;3(1): 105–112.

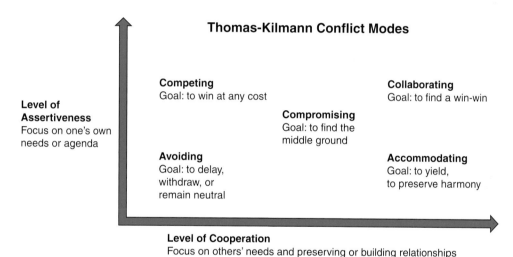

Thomas-Kilmann Conflict Modes

Fig. 6.2 The Thomas-Kilmann Conflict Modes describe an individual's predominant behavior during conflict. Although an individual may prefer one mode more commonly over others, a different mode may be more useful depending on context, including which mode is being used by other parties involved or what resources are available. (Adapted from Thomas KW. Conflict and conflict management. In: Dunnette, MD, ed. *Handbook of Industrial and Organizational Psychology.* Chicago: Rand McNally; 1976: 889–935.)

another[13] and as such can be used as a springboard for coaching conversations.

Physicians of tomorrow must serve as both informal and formal leaders and therefore need to develop skills such as executive presence, communication and relational skills, emotional intelligence, and time and team management. The Clifton Strengths Finder, Myers-Briggs, or Thomas-Kilmann (Fig. 6.2)[14] instruments can be used as frameworks to help learners and emerging faculty leaders become aware of their individual leadership styles and how their individual styles can be best used for change management or problem-solving in the system at large. Additionally, the Kane-Baltes Leadership Self-Efficacy Survey has specifically been developed to measure self-perceived capability as a team leader.[15] Use of the objective individualized data from these tools can be applied to teach and assess leadership skills in the context of several, if not all, of the ACGME competencies.

DEVELOPING EFFECTIVE EDUCATORS

Coaching can be an effective way to support the development of educators at any level, from medical students to practicing physicians. Teaching skills can be developed through informal social learning interactions such as peer-to-peer coaching or through a more formal educator development process using structured coach-coachee pairings.

Social learning opportunities, such as those experienced in a community of practice, can be a means for experienced and aspiring educators to develop and refine their skills together in a collaborative, informal, and self-directed environment. In a community of practice, the coach and coachee roles may be dynamic, and although one person might serve as a coach for one skillset, they may be a coachee for a skillset in which they are less familiar. Similarly, tools such as the R2C2 (Relationship, Reaction, Content, Coaching),[16] Peer-Assessment Debriefing Instrument,[17] or the Stanford Faculty Development Program framework for teaching effectiveness[18] can be used to guide peer-to-peer observation and coaching for educators wanting to improve their practice.

An emerging practice in medical education is the development of formal coaching programs aimed at developing teaching practices in novice educators. These programs are housed in professional societies such as the Council of Emergency Medicine Residency Directors or at the institutional or school level. They may also be embedded in a department or division. The coaches in more formalized programs have specific training on how to coach with coach-coachee pairings that are longitudinal over time.

PHYSICAL HEALTH AND EMOTIONAL WELL-BEING

Increasing attention is being given to the effect of physician well-being on patient outcomes and health care systems. Accrediting bodies such as the Liaison Committee on Medical Education (LCME) and ACGME require programs to help learners develop skills to support and manage their own well-being. So far, we have outlined myriad academic applications of coaching, but coaching tools and frameworks are also useful for fostering a proactive approach to self-care and health behavior change.

Studies have shown that professional coaching programs for physicians can decrease emotional exhaustion and burnout symptoms and improve resilience and professional well-being.[10,19,20] Prioritizing physical and emotional well-being consistently during the status quo equips coachees with the confidence and tools to thrive during times of increased stress and even model such behaviors for their patients and colleagues. As learners develop skills to make effective changes in their personal lives, they are building competence in creative problem-solving and, over time, a sense of resilience and self-efficacy.

When coachees feel physically well and mentally strong, they maintain a greater capacity to cope with physical and psychological challenges, such as experiencing loss and grief, that inevitably arise during their training and careers as physicians.

Over time, through consistent practice, coachees are creating a personalized toolkit and sustainable framework for thriving during challenges and improving long-term resilience. Practicing mindfulness, self-discovery, and self-compassion on a consistent basis empowers learners to approach personal and professional setbacks, including medical errors or unanticipated poor patient outcomes, with a growth mindset. Practicing mindfulness also enhances one's self-awareness and ability to self-regulate during times when emotions and stakes are highest, which ultimately cultivates higher emotional intelligence (Chapter 3).

MANAGING UNCERTAINTY AND DISRUPTIVE CHANGE

Maintaining health and well-being during times of personal stress and rapid change prepares learners to more effectively manage uncertainties and change in their professional lives. Uncertainty is ubiquitous to the human experience on a personal level, and it is specifically inherent to the medical profession, where trainees and attending physicians are often faced with diagnostic or treatment uncertainties in patient care. Furthermore, trainees are expected to adapt to change frequently when rotating with new teams of students, residents, and staff; shifting between disciplines; alternating from inpatient to outpatient venues; or sometimes working an overnight shift on the first day of a rotation in a new environment or discipline they have never experienced—all of which are routine occurrences in undergraduate medical training.

The expectation to rapidly transition continues as resident physicians move through different subspecialty rotations every 2 to 4 weeks and face uncertainty each time they progress into new roles with increasing responsibilities and autonomy (evolving from intern to junior and senior resident, chief resident or fellow, and eventually independent practitioner). Physicians entering independent practice similarly face uncertainty when accepting a job at a new institution, shifting to administrative or leadership roles, experiencing a change in leadership at their institution, adapting to hospital policies or coding regulations, and of course, personal and familial experiences that may alter their career trajectory.

Imposter phenomenon (sometimes referred to in the literature as imposter symptoms, imposterism, or imposter syndrome) is not uncommon in high-achieving individuals or those with high degrees of perfectionism, including physicians and health sciences trainees, and may be associated with psychological distress[21,22] or components of burnout.[23] Although self-doubt variably affects physicians, it is not limited to experiences during medical training and, in fact, can occur at any career stage.[24] Transitioning into a new role brings some level of uncertainty and possibly thoughts of self-doubt and fear of failure.

Early on, coaching teaches goal-setting skills to adapt to and, ideally, to proactively seek change and helps learners shift their focus to factors within their control rather than factors they cannot control. Skilled coaches encourage learners to embrace each challenge as an opportunity to master new skills with a mindful appreciation, creativity, and growth mindset. Positive change experiences ultimately equip coachees with individualized self-soothing techniques to appreciate and learn from their failures (rather than fear them) and to grow from their successes along the way.

Approaching uncertainty with creativity, curiosity, and exploration of new possibilities can help combat the anxieties and negative self-talk that accompany imposter syndrome. It is also paramount for coaches to support learners in practicing self-compassion during times of perceived failure or after errors occur. Over time, the self-discovery, coping skills, sense of mastery, and self-efficacy that evolves through coaching help learners maintain an internal locus of control during transitions, uncertainty, or instability in their environment.

DEVELOPING SKILLS IN SELF-DIRECTED LEARNING AND CHANGE

Medicine is changing exponentially. As such, there is increased emphasis on developing master adaptive learners who identify and mitigate their gaps in knowledge and skills. Previously, much of learning relied on the banking method where the "expert" imparts knowledge on the "novice." In the banking method, learners are passive participants in the learning process, and their learning activities are directed by their teacher.

Coaching seeks to shift the burden of knowledge acquisition from the teacher to the learner; whereas the learner identifies what they need to know along with associated learning strategies and resources. A coach supports the master adaptive learner and this self-directed learning process by facilitating informed self-assessment, providing individualized feedback on performance, and serving as a resource for the learner as they identify specific and actionable steps to take to achieve their learning goals.

We know from previous literature that unguided self-assessment can be inaccurate.[25] However, guided or informed self-assessment, a process by which a learner collects and analyzes internal and external data sources and compares them against a standard, can yield a more accurate appraisal of skills and knowledge.[26] Coaches play a pivotal role in the development of the skills needed to perform an informed self-assessment.

As previously described, physicians and those in training can experience imposter syndrome. By developing skills to perform an informed self-assessment, coaches can help learners improve their self-assessment accuracy, and this "reality check" is a crucial step in combating imposter symptoms. Although the coach's role will vary over time based on the acumen of the learner, they will help the learner determine the validity and appropriateness of data sources and the accuracy of the learner's interpretation of the collected data. Ultimately, the learner will develop the skills necessary to become a master adaptive learner in order to direct their own learning.

TAKE-HOME POINTS

1. Coaching is most effective when goals emerge from intrinsic motivators linked to personal values and long-term vision.
2. Coaching can be effective in addressing a variety of personal and professional goals ranging from health and well-being to specific professional skills development.
3. When mandated by program leadership, such as in remediation of core competencies, coaching is most effective when eliciting core values, strengths, and aspirations from the coachee and linking these to professional goals; goals are still driven by the learner, with coach guidance.
4. Coaching can help learners develop skills that support self-directed lifelong learning—and growing into master adaptive learners.

QUESTIONS FOR FURTHER THOUGHT

1. What resources are required to train someone to be an effective coach for the applications discussed in this chapter?
2. What resources are necessary to support the coaching process when coachees shift between learning venues, for example, from the classroom to various clinical settings?
3. How can coaching foster a culture that emphasizes growth mindset for learners while simultaneously prioritizing quality and safety outcomes?

ANNOTATED BIBLIOGRAPHY

Kalet A, Buckvar-Keltz L, Harnik V, et al. Measuring professional identity formation early in medical school. *Med Teach.* 2017;39(3):255–261.
Kalet and colleagues demonstrate the correlation of a tool, the professional identity essay (PIE), with established moral reasoning measures. Data from the PIE can be shared with medical students as a potential means to augment their professional identity formation.

Mangrulkar RS, Tsai A, Cox SM, et al. A proposed shared vision for leadership development for all medical students: a call from a coalition of diverse medical schools. *Teach Learn Med.* 2020 May 2:1–8.
Mangrulkar and colleagues discuss the importance of leadership development for all medical students and provide tools and a proposed framework for incorporating leadership training into medical education.

Moore M, Jackson E, Tschannen-Moran B, eds. *Coaching Psychology Manual.* 2nd ed. Philadelphia: Wolters Kluwer; 2016:71–92.
Moore and colleagues provide a manual for the principles and frameworks used in coaching and the science behind them. This practical guide demonstrates how specific coaching skills and tools can be applied to a diverse range of coaching scenarios.

Palamara K, Kauffman C, Stone VE, et al. Promoting success: A professional development coaching program for interns in medicine. *J Grad Med Educ.* 2015;7(4):630–637.
Palamara and colleagues describe their experience using the principles of positive psychology to develop an evidence-based professional development coaching program for medicine interns. Their findings highlight the positive reception to such programs from learners and the need to develop and provide ongoing training for coaches.

Reynolds AK. Academic coaching for learners in medical education: twelve tips for the learning specialist. *Med Teach.* 2020;42(6):616–621.
Reynolds uses literature from a variety of disciplines and his experiences as an educator to outline twelve tips for medical educators to develop their coaching competence. The tips help readers situate the learner as the expert in their own learning and are intended to support the promotion of lifelong learning.

REFERENCES

1. Lovell B. What do we know about coaching in medical education? A literature review. *Med Educ.* 2018;52(4):376–390.
2. Cooke M, Irby DM, O'Brien BC. *Educating Physicians: A Call for Reform of Medical School and Residency.* San Francisco: Jossey-Bass; 2010.
3. Bebeau MJ, Monson VE. Professional identity formation and transformation across the lifespan. In: McKee A, Eraut M, eds. *Learning Trajectories, Innovation and Identity in Professional Development.* Dordrecht, Netherlands: Springer; 2012:135–162.
4. Kalet A, Buckvar-Keltz L, Harnik V, Monson V, Hubbard S, Crowe R, Song HS, Yingling S. Measuring professional identity formation early in medical school. *Med Teach.* 2017 Mar;39(3):255–261.
5. Deiorio NM, Carney PA, Kahl LE, Bonura EM, Juve AM. Coaching: a new model for academic and career achievement. *Med Educ Online.* 2016;21(1):33480.
6. Ericsson KA. Deliberate practice and the acquisition and maintenance of expert performance in medicine and related domains. *Acad Med.* 2004;79(10 suppl):S70–S81.
7. Reynolds AK. Academic coaching for learners in medical education: twelve tips for the learning specialist. *Med Teach.* 2020;42(6):616–621.
8. Moore M, Jackson E, Tschannen-Moran B. *Coaching Psychology Manual.* 2nd ed. Philadelphia: Wolters Kluwer; 2016:71–92.
9. Lucey C, Souba W. Perspective: the problem with the problem of professionalism. *Acad Med.* 2010 June;85(6):1018–1024.
10. Palamara K, Kauffman C, Stone VE, et al. Promoting success: A professional development coaching program for interns in medicine. *J Grad Med Educ.* 2015;7(4):630–637.
11. Iserson KV. Talking about professionalism through the lens of professional identity. *AEM Educ Train.* 2018;3(1):105–112.
12. Rotenstein LS, Sadun R, Jena AB. Why doctors need leadership training. *Harvard Business Review.* Oct 17, 2018.
13. Mangrulkar RS, Tsai A, Cox SM, et al. A proposed shared vision for leadership development for all medical students: a call from a coalition of diverse medical schools. *Teach Learn Med.* 2020 May 2:1–8.
14. Thomas KW. Conflict and conflict management. In: Dunnette MD, ed. *Handbook of Industrial and Organizational Psychology.* Chicago: Rand McNally; 1976:889–935.

15. Chao C, Wooten K, Spratt H, et al. Integration of leadership training for graduate and medical students engaged in translational biomedical research: examining self-efficacy and self-insight. *J Clin Transl Sci.* 2018;2(1):48–52.

16. Sargeant J, Lockyer J, Mann K, et al. Facilitated reflective performance feedback: developing an evidence- and theory-based model that builds relationship, explores reactions and content, and coaches for performance change (R2C2). *Acad Med.* 2015;90(12):1698–1706.

17. Saylor JL, Wainwright SF, Herge EA, Pohlig RT. Peer-assessment debriefing instrument (PADI): assessing faculty effectiveness in simulation education. *J Allied Health.* 2016;45(3):e27–e30.

18. Mintz M, Southern DA, Ghali WA, Ma IW. Validation of the 25-item Stanford Faculty Development Program Tool on clinical teaching effectiveness. *Teach Learn Med.* 2015;27(2):174–181.

19. Dyrbye LN, Shanafelt TD, Gill PR, et al. Effect of a professional coaching intervention on the well-being and distress of physicians: a pilot randomized clinical trial. *JAMA Intern Med.* 2019;179(10):1406–1414.

20. McGonagle AK, Schwab L, Yahanda N, et al. Coaching for primary care physician well-being: A randomized trial and follow-up analysis. *J Occup Health Psychol.* 2020;25(5):297–314.

21. Henning K, Ey S, Shaw D. Perfectionism, the imposter phenomenon and psychological adjustment in the medical, dental, nursing, and pharmacy students. *Med Educ.* 1998;32(5):456–464.

22. Oriel K, Plane MB, Mundt M. Family medicine residents and the impostor phenomenon. *Fam Med.* 2004;36(4):248–252.

23. Villwock JA, Sobin LB, Koester LA, Harris TM. Impostor syndrome and burnout among American medical students: a pilot study. *Int J Med Educ.* 2016;7:364–369.

24. LaDonna KA, Ginsburg S, Watling C. Rising to the level of your incompetence:" what physicians' self-assessment of their performance reveals about the imposter syndrome in medicine. *Acad Med.* 2018;93(5):763–768.

25. Eva KW, Cunnington JP, Reiter HI, et al. How can I know what I don't know? Poor self assessment in a well-defined domain. *Adv Health Sci Educ Theory Pract.* 2004;9(3): 211–224.

26. Mann K, van der Vleuten C, Eva K, et al. Tensions in informed self-assessment: how the desire for feedback and reticence to collect and use it can conflict. *Acad Med.* 2011;86(9):1120–1127.

7

Coaching for Performance Improvement

Indira Bhavsar-Burke, Rishindra M. Reddy, Maya M. Hammoud, and Kimberly D. Lomis

LEARNING OBJECTIVES

1. Apply coaching techniques to support improved learner performance in clinical reasoning.
2. Describe the relationship between clinical reasoning and the development of master adaptive learners.
3. Recognize when content expertise is needed in coaching the master adaptive learner.
4. Describe the application of coaching for improving performance in procedural settings and addressing cognitive, technical, and communication skills.

CHAPTER OUTLINE

CHAPTER SUMMARY

This chapter describes the role of coaching to improve performance in clinical reasoning and to support the development of master adaptive learners. We review the theoretical framework of clinical reasoning, including specific domains of clinical reasoning that improve with coaching. Lastly, we outline the application of content expertise in coaching for procedural settings, addressing cognitive skills, technical performance, and communication skills.

INTRODUCTION

Coaching is a useful tool to guide learners longitudinally throughout their careers. Its focus on self-awareness and intrinsic motivation is critical to its ongoing success, ensuring learners prioritize opportunities and career advancement in accordance with an overarching vision. Arming learners with the skills to adjust to change becomes paramount as the landscape of medical education shifts and learners are forced to more frequently adapt to new environments and advances in health care.

Master adaptive learners possess the skills necessary to demonstrate continuous improvement through learning. The Master Adaptive Learner model is a metacognitive approach in which self-reflection and adaptive practice are used to foster learning and promote learner success. It is discussed in more detail in Chapter 2 of this handbook. Master adaptive learners use a framework of iterative adjustments founded in the principles of improving performance to address gaps in medical knowledge, patient care, and clinical decision-making. They employ a systems-based approach to learning based on humble inquiry, best available evidence, teamwork, motivation, communication, and feedback. A strong foundation in clinical reasoning and skills development empowers the master adaptive learner to meet challenges proactively in clinical practice.

Vignette

AB is a first-year general surgery resident who is consulted on a 45-year-old woman admitted to the medicine service with biliary pancreatitis. The patient improves and is discharged home but is later readmitted to the intensive care unit with a recurrent attack. AB correctly identified that the patient would ultimately require cholecystectomy but failed to recognize the risk of a recurrent gallbladder attack if she were discharged without follow-up. AB forgot to communicate this to the patient and did not include it in the discharge recommendations in the electronic health record.

Thought Questions

1. How could coaching help AB recognize this mistake and prevent it in the future?
2. Can improved clinical reasoning skills decrease these types of errors?

Coaching helps learners identify areas of improvement so that they are better equipped to recognize opportunities for continuous skills development. Coaching for performance improvement in medical education is inherently different from coaching for career development. It is a cyclical process that mirrors that of the Master Adaptive Learner model described by Cutrer and colleagues.[1] It relies heavily on deliberate practice in which careful attention is paid to repetitive practice, reflection, and identification of future goals. Coaching for performance improvement relies on the role of content expertise—coaches in this setting must possess the skills they intend to cultivate in their learners for coaching to be effective.

In this chapter, we discuss the significance of clinical reasoning in the development of the master adaptive learner and the utility of coaching in creating a foundation for strong clinical reasoning skills. We also discuss the application of performance and skills improvement in the field of surgical coaching to develop technical performance and communication skills.

UNDERSTANDING CLINICAL REASONING IN THE CONTEXT OF THE MASTER ADAPTIVE LEARNER

Iterative learning is central to the aims of the master adaptive learner. Development of reasoning skills and thoughtful medical decision-making are necessary to promote adaptive learning and are best reinforced for learners using specific educational theories. To address the roles

of clinical reasoning and the need for content expertise in performance coaching, we describe these theories briefly in this chapter. Discussing these theories openly with learners during the coaching process has been shown to improve self-awareness and aid in clinical performance.[2]

Dual Process Theory

Dual process theory has been adapted from the psychology literature to help explain the ways in which clinicians arrive at medical decisions. It was made popular by Daniel Kahneman's book, *Thinking Fast and Slow*. Decisions are made via two cognitive pathways called System 1 (thinking fast) and System 2 (thinking slow).[2]

System 1 is intuitive and automatic; experts spend most of their time reasoning through clinical cases via System 1. They analyze situations quickly and compare their current experience with past experiences using illness scripts and preexisting medical knowledge. In contrast, System 2 is more logical and analytical; novices spend much of their time approaching clinical cases through System 2 reasoning. In individual scenarios, the pathway in which a case is considered is based on the prior experience of the learner.

Appropriate diagnosis and clinical management depend on adequate and frequent transitions between the two systems. Master adaptive learners use System 2 to check the diagnoses they arrive at using System 1. Failure to recognize the roles of Systems 1 and 2 in clinical reasoning and decision-making frequently leads to diagnostic errors, such as preliminary anchoring bias. Understanding dual process theory empowers learners to approach clinical cases with the goals of improving clinical performance and problem-solving skills, as well as the development of clinical expertise.

Cognitive Load Theory

Cognitive load theory is central to the concepts of clinical reasoning and problem-solving skills. It refers to the number of resources available in a learner's working memory at a given time. Generally, individuals can process seven +/− two items in their working memory but their long-term memory is essentially limitless. Additionally, retrieval of information from long-term memory is effortless whereas reliance on working memory is fraught with limitations, such as processing speed and overall capacity.[3]

As learners transition from novices to experts, they can coordinate more information in their working memories in the form of illness scripts. This allows learners to engage with increasing amounts of clinical information without overwhelming their working memories and to draw on past experiences to inform their current decision making.

Decision-making in clinical practice is often complex—it requires learners to critically appraise situations and

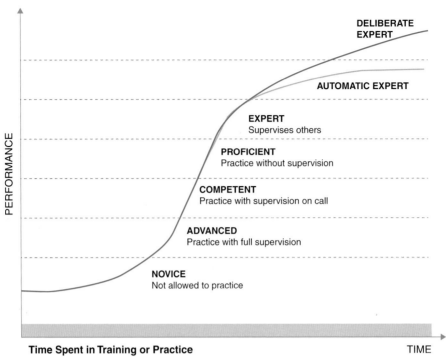

Fig. 7.1 Clinical reasoning and performance development of the master adaptive learner through deliberate practice. (Kalet A, Pusic M. Defining and assessing competence. In: Kalet A, Chou C, eds. *Remediation in Medical Education.* Boston: Springer; 2014:3–15.)

modify their decisions based on the best available evidence. Cognitive load theory is an important consideration in the development of the master adaptive learner; it allows learners to engage with a larger breadth of clinical data when making important medical decisions.

Deliberate Practice Theory

The concept of deliberate practice is the foundation by which novices become experts. Its focus is primarily on the cultivation of expertise, which is founded on the belief that experts are created through repeated and deliberate practice over an extensive length of time. It is easy to see how the concept of deliberate practice applies to medical training, which is based on years of extensive study and practical application throughout medical school and residency training.[4]

Deliberate practice states that experience alone is not enough to create expertise. Experts are created not just through repetition of a particular skill but through deliberate practice of the components of that skill coupled with feedback on performance. This becomes increasingly important in technical and procedural coaching, as well as complex medical decision-making. Deliberate practice and the development of expertise relies heavily on a self-reflective

feedback loop that is central to the formation of the master adaptive learner. It promotes the model of lifelong learning; deliberate experts can make iterative adjustments to adapt throughout the course of their careers despite medical advancements and changes within the health care system.

Figure 7.1 provides a schematic for coaches to share with learners, outlining the process of deliberate practice and the development of competence within medical decision-making and improving technical skills. Coaches may engage learners in exercises in deliberate practice to foster self-awareness and empower motivation for personal improvement.

COACHING FOR PERFORMANCE IMPROVEMENT IN CLINICAL REASONING

Self-directed learning is a concept inherent to the Master Adaptive Learner model. Successful self-directed learning occurs when individuals can identify knowledge gaps, develop goals to address those gaps, improve their performance, and reflect on the process to discover further potential areas for progress. In many cases, however, learners are ill-equipped to identify their own areas of improvement. In these scenarios, unguided self-assessment is unlikely to be beneficial for learners who may ultimately require feedback from a content expert to identify areas of potential growth.

Coaching is a highly individualized process that depends on both the nature of the learner and the skills and experience of the coach. Successful coaching relationships require commitment from both parties and a mutual understanding of the learner's goals. When learners struggle to formulate goals or fail to recognize areas of improvement, coaches with content expertise can bridge the gap. Content expertise allows a coach to pinpoint the learner's potential areas of improvement and empowers them to set goals as a team. This is particularly useful in coaching medical decision-making, surgical or technical skills, and communication.

Research has shown that content expertise is essential to coach learners who struggle with clinical performance and complex medical decision-making.[1] In general, content experts are specially equipped to identify the learner's areas of improvement, which usually occur in one of five domains: data collection, hypothesis generation, problem representation, knowledge organization, or assessment and treatment (Fig. 7.2). For coaching to be successful, adequate observation of the learner in real-time clinical environments is crucial so that appropriate identification of deficits can be made.

Data Collection

Learners who are unable to gather information at the bedside and/or use appropriate channels of communication to collect data may struggle with clinical performance. Early learners who require coaching in data collection are often identified by disembodied interviewing rather than hypothesis-driven interviewing; students may ask random questions during a clinical encounter without tailoring them to a specific differential diagnosis. Advanced learners who struggle with data collection may not be able to communicate effectively with other services. Oftentimes, this is identified as a lack of awareness regarding when to request consultations or an inability to recognize the importance of nursing updates and overnight clinical events in the context of a particular clinical scenario. Challenges with navigating electronic health records (EHRs) are also common. Learners may experience difficulties synthesizing data from the EHR in the context of a particular patient or may become overwhelmed with the large volume of historical data maintained in the EHR. These difficulties commonly manifest as issues with efficiency and organization.

In many ways, data collection is the foundation by which medical decisions are made. Without direct observation and feedback from a content expert, many learners are unable to identify data collection as an area of potential improvement. Luckily, coaches can employ a variety of tools to hone this skill over time through ongoing deliberate practice. Data collection skills improve with exercises in which learners are coached to generate differential diagnoses before a clinical encounter, allowing them to tailor their interview to the most plausible medical ailments. Challenging learners to report a limited list of no more than five objective data points (such as laboratory values or imaging results) promotes focused data collection and enables learners to identify salient information more readily.

Data collection is also a skill required for the development of the master adaptive learner; it is not only useful in clinical practice but also in the personal growth and advancement of the learner. Master adaptive learners develop critical thinking skills by considering information in a series of phases: planning, learning, assessing, and adjusting. Data collection is especially important in the *planning* phase of the master adaptive learner process. In this phase, learners can identify opportunities for learning in the context of their personal experience to address potential knowledge gaps. This is often done through thoughtful questioning, in which learners examine situations from different perspectives. Deliberate practice to improve data collection will ultimately help improve both clinical performance and personal identification of areas of growth.

Problem Representation

Problem representation refers to the process of identifying key features of clinical scenarios. In general, it refers to the learner's ability to identify who the patient is, the time

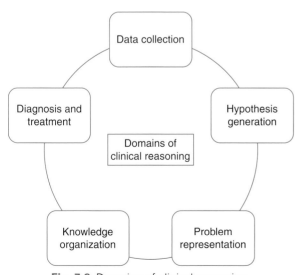

Fig. 7.2 Domains of clinical reasoning.

course of the patient's illness, and the most likely illness or clinical syndrome with which the patient is presenting. Successful problem representation can only occur if learners are able to adequately collect data. Early learners who struggle with problem representation may not be equipped to distinguish salient details from extraneous ones; they are often identified as not being able to "see the forest for the trees." Advanced learners who struggle with problem representation may understand which objective data is clinically relevant but lack the skills necessary to link that information to a clinical syndrome.

Problem representation requires learners to prioritize the information they obtain in clinical practice in real time. It requires consistent and constant reframing, an exercise that is commonly used in coaching to improve clinical performance in this domain. Learners must recognize that problem representations are fluid and change as new information is discovered. Improved problem representation occurs when learners reassess clinical scenarios as more objective data is available. As patients progress through a hospital admission, for example, the problem representation changes as the patient transitions from the emergency department to the ward and again based on the trajectory of the patient's illness throughout the hospital admission. Coaches should challenge learners to present an updated one-line summary of the patient each time the patient is discussed on rounds to promote reframing and prevent anchoring bias.

In many ways, problem representation is akin to the iterative learning process of the master adaptive learner. Once learners have identified knowledge gaps, they must then prioritize their approach to addressing these gaps. This can only occur if learners are prepared to consider new information as it becomes available to reorder their priorities for learning based on ongoing needs assessments.

Hypothesis Generation

Once learners are equipped to appropriately gather data and describe its significance, they must then analyze the data within the scaffolding of their clinical experience to generate a list of differential diagnoses. Hypothesis generation relies heavily on dual process theory, which describes the interplay between nonanalytic and analytic clinical reasoning. Early learners who struggle with hypothesis generation may not be able to recognize more than typical presentations of common diseases. Similarly, they may focus more on common presentations of uncommon diseases as opposed to uncommon presentations of common diseases. Advanced learners who struggle with hypothesis generation may display inappropriate anchoring bias or rely heavily on pattern recognition, forgetting to toggle between Systems 1 and 2 when considering clinical cases.

Coaching is a useful modality for addressing deficits in hypothesis generation. Methods to improve performance in hypothesis generation include frequent clinical "what if" questions to reflect on how new information changes the existing clinical scenario. Hypothesis generation improves when learners are coached to consider how changes in patient characteristics or symptoms affect potential diagnoses. Coaches are instructed to ask "what if" questions that then allow learners to consider how new information changes the differential diagnosis. For example, a patient presents to the clinic with shortness of breath. The differential is quite broad, but targeted questions like "What if the patient has a fever?" or "What if the patient has chest pain?" encourages learners to generate hypotheses more readily. This practice provides learners with the opportunity to reorganize their thoughts, ask themselves "what if" questions, and reflect on their prior decision-making.

Like data collection, hypothesis generation is also a critical element in the development of the master adaptive learner. For learners, this mirrors the act of generating an initial differential diagnosis. Once the initial prioritization has taken place, learners must then be able to recognize how new information may prompt them to reorder their priorities. Thoughtful coaching of hypothesis generation will allow learners to readily identify when adjustments need to be made, both in the process of patient care and during one's career.

Knowledge Organization

Knowledge organization is an essential tool in clinical medicine and the basis by which clinicians consider the data they have amassed to make medical decisions. Appropriate knowledge organization requires learners to adequately collect data and generate a differential. Once learners can do this, they can then consider their generated differential diagnoses in the form of illness scripts. Understanding cognitive load theory is important when considering knowledge organization. Early learners who struggle with knowledge organization may only be able to identify a short list of possible diagnoses because they have not yet been exposed to a broader breadth of clinical scenarios. Advanced learners who struggle with knowledge organization are often cited as being disorganized or inefficient.

Coaching is an effective tool for improving knowledge organization. This skill can be developed by dedicated study of symptomatology as opposed to different disease states. This gives learners the opportunity to consider clinical scenarios in the context of the presenting symptoms, enabling them to work toward a diagnosis as opposed to considering a diagnosis and working backward to see if the patient is exhibiting the associated symptoms.

The skills one develops in knowledge organization are again critical to the development of the master adaptive learner. In many ways, the ability to organize knowledge and work toward a diagnosis requires a similar skillset needed by learners to prioritize goal advancement. Learners who excel in knowledge organization are more successful in pursuing goals without being overwhelmed by details and extraneous information. They are better equipped to search for information and consider new opportunities because they have an existing framework by which to catalog new data.

Assessment and Treatment

The last domain of clinical reasoning and performance development is assessment and treatment. Once learners have generated a list of possible diagnoses and organized the differential within the framework of their clinical experience, they are ready to engage in medical decision-making. Early learners who struggle with disease management are unable to arrive at the correct diagnosis; usually this is a result of poor knowledge organization and lack of clinical experience. Advanced learners who struggle with assessment and treatment may not be able to understand the severity of the underlying disease and are unable to enact detailed treatment plans beyond the initial work-up. In many cases, learner hesitancy due to a lack of confidence, or in severe cases imposter syndrome, can manifest as difficulty in assessment and treatment.

Content expertise is imperative for coaching medical decision-making, as it requires familiarity with commonly encountered disease states and allows learners to engage in "if, then" decision-making in a controlled environment. Assessment and treatment skills can be coached most effectively by external feedback and self-reflection. Successful coaching of medical decision-making relies on learners' abilities to experiment with their treatment plans, so they gain both the necessary skills needed for clinical performance and improved confidence. As learners become experts, they are able to use feedback, in the form of clinical data, to determine whether their treatments are working, which will then prompt them to adjust their treatment plans if necessary. Learner hesitancy often improves with simulation exercises that help identify whether learners have gaps in medical knowledge or lack confidence. For example, simulation exercises in which learners are at the bedside of a decompensating patient with mock codes empower learners to make decisions in a safe environment so they feel comfortable doing the same in clinical practice.

The concepts that are reinforced by coaching medical decision-making are the same concepts that master adaptive learners use in the *assessing* phase of learning. Master adaptive learners rely on both self-assessment and external feedback to identify knowledge gaps and determine whether their learning is adequate for the gap they are working to address. Development of critical thinking skills and self-reflection are essential and must occur simultaneously for learning to be successful, both in clinical practice and career advancement.

APPLICATION OF COACHING TO PROCEDURAL SETTINGS

Coaching technical and procedural skills requires content expertise and relies on the development of strong clinical reasoning and communication skills. Procedural education occurs in many arenas, sometimes in formal didactic lectures, but usually in more informal settings with one-on-one or one-on-two types of interactions.[4] These informal sessions have a different focus than formalized teaching sessions based on a set curriculum, but include aspects of teaching, coaching, and mentoring. Coaching embodies some aspects of teaching and mentoring but differentiates itself by focusing on the improvement of existing skills, rather than the teaching of new skills. Mentoring is similarly different in that it is even less structured and not focused on specific skills or performance.[5] Coaching tends to be the key interaction in the procedural settings. Procedural coaches need to be highly respected content experts, have strong communication and interpersonal skills, be active listeners, and be able to adapt their approach based on their learners' needs.[5]

The operating room or procedural suite is a unique environment that is focused first and foremost on patient care. Although serving to lead the actual execution of a procedure, these coaches are simultaneously addressing the needs of multiple levels of learners, such as medical students, residents, and fellows. Procedural coaches multitask to create safe environments for both patient care and learning. Learners perceive coaches as effective when they exhibit joy for teaching, encourage independent learning, and foster open communication.[4] Effective coaches embody many of the attributes of the master adaptive learner described earlier in this chapter, including independent learning, humble inquiry, and self-reflection. Procedural coaching must address cognitive, technical, and communication skills. In addition to cultivating these skills, coaches must also model these behaviors to serve as a positive example but also to gain credibility with their learners and other team members.

Table 7.1 provides examples of modeling, teaching, and coaching performance-based skills. Learners rely on the content expertise of coaches. In addition to surgical expertise, communication and critical reasoning skills are key

TABLE 7.1   Examples of Modeling, Teaching, and Coaching Performance-Based Skills

	Modeling	Coaching	Teaching
Cognitive skills	• Determining the need for procedural intervention and deciding appropriate technical approach • Reviewing relevant clinical information and imaging prior to and during the procedure • Discussing any unique patient factors that may affect the risk of complications during or after the procedure	• Exploring a learner's understanding of patient information and indications for procedure • Probing the learner to consider alternative scenarios • Encouraging a trainee to anticipate procedural challenges and consider alternative plans • Structured debriefing after mock oral examinations	• Didactic lectures, curriculum based • Mock oral exams if focused on specific topics • Teaching history and physicals or presentation skills in a formalized manner
Technical skills	• Demonstrating proper techniques • Discussing potential alternative techniques • Describing level of satisfaction with the results of specific steps of the procedure	• Providing appropriate opportunities for supervised practice • Giving specific, actionable feedback on skills	• Didactic curriculum around technical skills • Simulation curricula
Communication skills	• Leading or discussing shared decision-making and process of obtaining patient consent • Communicating clearly and empathetically with the patient • Communicating effectively with other team members (e.g., technical staff, colleagues) and actively inviting the input of other team members throughout the procedure • Demonstrating leadership during formal time out and other critical points of the operation requiring communication (transition points, emergent scenarios)	• Explicitly addressing trainee communication skills (speaking respectfully and clearly to the patient and to other team members) • Commenting on learner's response to feedback or to the input of other team members during procedure • For residents, preparing them to assume a leadership role when faculty step out and providing guidance about when to ask for assistance	• Team training activities • Formal simulation-based communication skills training

elements of the patient care cycle that coaches must exhibit to develop a safe learning environment. There are multiple potential frameworks that can be used to coach these skills, some of which are discussed in practical terms in this chapter.

The Coaching in Medicine model, described by Rassbach and Blankenburg, is a continuous performance improvement model based on the principles of growth mindset, reflective practice, self-determination theory, lifelong learning, and goal setting.[6,7] The model emphasizes

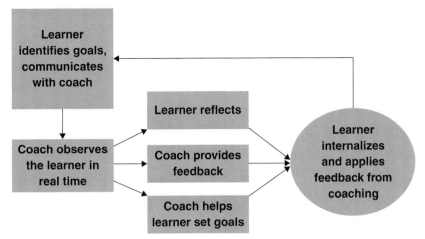

Fig. 7.3 Coaching in medicine conceptual model.

a relationship between the learner and the coach that is grounded in psychological safety, mutual trust, and vulnerability. As illustrated in Figure 7.3, each coaching session begins with the learner reflecting on their own strengths, weaknesses, and goals and sharing those reflections with a trusted coach. The coach then observes the learner in real time in a clinical setting for anywhere from minutes to hours, depending on the learner's goals. After the observation, the coach asks the learner to reflect on their performance, specifically what went well, what did not go well, and what questions arose. The coach then provides feedback to the learner based on the learner's reflections and on the coach's observations. The learner and coach work together to identify next steps and future goals for what the learner can work on and how the coach can help support the learner's growth. Finally, the learner incorporates the feedback and reflections from the coaching session to apply and practice in future clinical encounters.

The R2C2 framework was developed by Sargeant et al.[8] as a framework to facilitate feedback using a coaching approach. The R2C2 framework includes four phases: (1) building a relationship; (2) exploring reactions (to the feedback); (3) exploring content (of the feedback); and (4) coaching for performance change. This evidence- and theory-informed framework is based on elements that enhance recipients' engagement with, acceptance of, and productive use of feedback and has been studied in multiple specialties.[8-10]

Coaching in the operating room can employ this type of framework, but the traditional method of scheduling students on rotations may need to be modified to allow for optimal coaching. Students need time with their teachers to build the relationship, which may be better accomplished

through a day spent together in clinic rather than first introductions occurring in the operating room. Once this trust is built, the learner can better receive feedback and then make modifications in future practice. Graduate learners, who usually have longer-term relationships with faculty, may not need this same type of relationship building, but still need to have a strong foundation by which to receive feedback.

The R2C2 method for providing feedback in a coaching relationship also mirrors the iterative processes of the master adaptive learner. Once the coaching relationship is created, learners explore the feedback they receive in the same way master adaptive learners engage in the *planning* phase of learning. Coaching for performance change allows learners to then use feedback in routine practice, adjusting their behaviors based on their coaching interactions. Successful application of the R2C2 method is based on strong clinical reasoning skills and appropriate analysis of existing data (data collection), identification of learning gaps (hypothesis generation), reasoned prioritization of next steps (knowledge organization), and suitable application of feedback to improve performance (assessment and treatment).[11]

Coaching for clinical performance extends beyond the technical skills learned in the operating room. It includes the complete cycle of clinical care, from history taking and medical decision-making to procedures and appropriate follow-up and communication with patients and colleagues. Learners are best able to care for patients and improve clinical performance if coaches are adept at providing feedback in all realms of clinical practice. Faculty development will need to be improved to develop physicians to be better coaches in the future.

TAKE-HOME POINTS

1. Effective coaching of clinical reasoning skills improves clinical care and promotes lifelong and self-directed learning.
2. Content expertise is required to effectively coach technical skills and improve clinical performance.
3. Coaching models are helpful tools to promote skills development in the master adaptive learner.

QUESTIONS FOR FURTHER THOUGHT

1. How do challenges in clinical reasoning affect clinical performance?
2. What tools can be used to successfully coach clinical performance across the spectrum of patient care responsibilities, including direct patient care and professionalism and communication?

ANNOTATED BIBLIOGRAPHY

Cutrer WB, Miller B, Pusic MV, et al. Fostering the development of master adaptive learners: a conceptual model to guide skill acquisition in medical education. *Acad Med.* 2017;92:70–75.
The master adaptive learner model is described in detail in this article. It can be used as a guide for coaches and learners alike to identify areas for potential growth and develop plans for performance improvement.

Ericsson KA. Deliberate practice and the acquisition and maintenance of expert performance in medicine and related domains. *Acad Med.* 2004;79:S70–S81.
This article identifies the role of deliberate practice in skills development and performance in medical education.

Szulewski A, Howes D, van Merriënboer JJG, Sweller J. From theory to practice: the application of cognitive load theory to the practice of medicine. *Acad Med.* 2021;96:24–30.
This article describes the role of cognitive load in medical education and helps coaches identify unnecessarily increased cognitive load among learners. It also provides a framework by which coaches can help learners catalog this information and improve their performance skills as a result.

REFERENCES

1. Cutrer WB, Miller B, Pusic MV, et al. Fostering the development of master adaptive learners: a conceptual model to guide skill acquisition in medical education. *Acad Med.* 2017;92:70–75.
2. Parsons AS, Wijesekera TP, Rencic JJ. The management script: a practical tool for teaching management reasoning. *Acad Med.* 2020;95:1179–1185.
3. Szulewski A, Howes D, van Merriënboer JJG, Sweller J. From theory to practice: the application of cognitive load theory to the practice of medicine. *Acad Med.* 2021;96:24–30.
4. Ericsson KA. Deliberate practice and the acquisition and maintenance of expert performance in medicine and related domains. *Acad Med.* 2004;79:S70–S81.
5. Sloan DA, Donnelly MB, Schwartz RW. The surgical clerkship: characteristics of the effective teacher. *Med Educ.* 1996;30(1):18–23.
6. Lin J, Reddy RM. Teaching, mentorship, and coaching in surgical education. *Thorac Surg Clin.* 2019;29(3):311–320.
7. Rassbach CE, Blankenburg R. A novel pediatric residency coaching program: outcomes after one year. *Acad Med.* 2018;93:430–434.
8. Sargeant J, Lockyer J, Mann K, et al. Facilitated reflective performance feedback: developing an evidence-and theory-based model that builds relationship, explores reactions and content, and coaches for performance change (R2C2). *Acad Med.* 2015;90:1698–1706.
9. Sargeant J, Lockyer JM, Mann K, et al. The R2C2 model in residency education: how does it foster coaching and promote feedback use? *Acad Med.* 2018;93:1055–1063.
10. Sargeant J, Mann K, Manos S, et al. R2C2 in action: testing an evidence-based model to facilitate feedback and coaching in residency. *JGME.* 2017;9:165–170.
11. Lockyer J, Armson H, Könings KD, et al. In-the-moment feedback and coaching: improving R2C2 for a new context. *JGME.* 2020;12:27–35.

8

Coaching and Ethics, Diversity, Equity, and Inclusion

Atul Agarwal, Binata Mukherjee, Mark Meyer, and Kimberly D. Lomis

LEARNING OBJECTIVES

1. Define ethical principles in the context of coaching.
2. Recognize inequities that may exist for learners from groups underrepresented in medicine.
3. Discuss considerations in coaching a diverse group of learners.
4. Recognize the ubiquity of bias and its structural basis.
5. Describe the importance of self-awareness in overcoming bias.

CHAPTER OUTLINE

CHAPTER SUMMARY

As coaching programs are introduced into medical education, both at the undergraduate and graduate levels, knowledge and utilization of ethical codes in coaching becomes essential. Adherence to these ethical standards is important in addressing inequities and promoting diversity and inclusion.

Recognizing that inequities exist in education, including medical education, coaches can be crucial to bridging the gap that learners from groups who are marginalized in medicine may experience. Effective coaching can draw upon the coachee's own strengths and resilience to help position them for success.

To support efforts to increase the representation and enhance the experience of groups historically and currently marginalized in medicine, coaching programs should focus on building a culture of mutual inclusivity and respect, where all participants feel welcomed and differences are valued. Coaches are in an ideal position to build this culture by developing structural competency and understanding how socialization contributes to bias. Through professional development activities, coaches can become aware of their own biases and become acquainted with the key tenets of ethics as they pertain to coaching.

INTRODUCTION

Adherence to ethical standards is incumbent to any coaching relationship. Intrinsic to coaching is the concept of contextual awareness as it applies to interacting with a diverse group of people that includes those from different privileges, backgrounds, beliefs, ways of expression, and life experiences. Faculty development in learning how to honor these differences by gaining insights into coaches' own unconscious biases and habits is unquestionably needed before initiating a coaching program and for maintenance of a program and an individual coach's skills.

COACHING AND ETHICS

Collaborative partnerships like those between a teacher and student, physician and patient, or any professional service provider and client share one common thread—they are vulnerable to a power differential between the individuals involved. Although the relationship between a coach and a coachee in noneducational settings may not involve any power differential, one definitely exists in academic medical settings. Therefore it is important that these interactions be governed by established ethical standards of behavior. Ram Ramanathan reminds us that "the responsibility to uphold coaching ethics is with the coach by establishing personal standards of ethics at a much higher level than what the profession calls for."[1]

The profession of medicine holds close scrutiny over its members and their professional qualifications. However, no such scrutiny is routinely enforced in coaching relationships; therefore, in the context of medical education, standardization is foundational, and individuals

---

Vignette 1

Anna is a rising third-year resident in internal medicine. As her coach, you have known Anna for over a year. When you first met her, you found her to be accomplished, highly motivated, and focused. You now find her more irritable, disinterested in her studies, and often unkempt. You decide to ask her directly how she is doing. She admits to a personal family matter that has been weighing on her for several months. She says she has been struggling to cope and knows she doesn't seem to be herself anymore. Upon further exploration, you find out she has been abusing alcohol and notice behaviors that could represent early signs of depression. Much to your dismay, her academic performance of late has followed suit.

Thought Questions

1. Which ethical principles surface based on changes in Anna's mental, physical, and academic standing?
2. How do these principles interact to raise ethical dilemmas for you as her coach?
3. What are some decision-making frameworks that you can rely on as a coach to "do the right thing?"

---

must abide by institutionally established ethical codes. To enhance uniformity, equity, and inclusivity, monitoring of the program's outcomes is necessary. Compliance with the established requirements ensures there are no unintended consequences among learners—in particular, those from underrepresented groups.

ETHICAL STANDARDS GOVERNING THE COACHING OF MEDICAL LEARNERS

Several professional coaching organizations have developed ethical guidelines: the International Coaching Federation,[2] International Association of Coaching,[3] Association for Coaching,[4] International Coaching Community,[5] and American Psychological Association,[6] with others such as the Institute of Coaching[7] following suit or subscribing to the guidelines of these major organizations. It is important to note that these are general guidelines. They are not legally binding and thus far are not under the jurisdiction of a governing body.

Although these organizations each have their own guidelines, they have commonalities that are worth focusing on. The ethical standard of "responsibility to clients" specifically asks a coach to manage power differences that may be caused by cultural or contextual issues. In education, this can apply to working with all learners, and coaches should be particularly mindful that learners from some groups experience a greater power differential. The "responsibility to practice and performance" standard seeks for the coach to commit to excellence through personal, professional, and ethical development. In the context of diversity, this can be done by becoming more aware of biases through continuous training. The standard concerning "responsibility to professionalism" holds the coach responsible for setting appropriate boundaries that are culturally sensitive. Finally, the "responsibility to society" standard seeks to avoid discrimination on the basis of age, race, gender expression, ethnicity, sexual orientation, religion, national origin, disability, or military status. This standard can be directly applied to improving inclusion in medical education.[2]

A coach looking for general ethical guidelines to abide by would be well served by referring to the following short-list of guidelines that are shared across several disciplines.[8] The first ethical guideline is akin to the Hippocratic oath of doing no harm. The second asks the coach to act to prioritize the welfare of others. The third reminds us not to practice dangerously by exceeding the limits of our knowledge. Finally, coaches are urged to honor the client's wishes and obey relevant laws, such as the Family Educational Rights and Privacy Act that protects the privacy of student education records. Passmore further describes the following as the main themes that can emerge in coaching: utility, autonomy, truth, confidentiality, avoiding harm, justice, and respecting the rights of others.[9]

COMMON ETHICAL DILEMMAS

Passmore et al. remind us that differences in how the various coaching organizations prioritize their guidelines may contribute to "cognitive dissonance." Coaches may be caught between two opposing values or principles and not know which ones to prioritize. These ethical dilemmas can stem from the coach or coachee, with either crossing the boundary; issues involving other individuals in an organization; or a combination thereof.[10]

The themes listed by Passmore must be highlighted in the context of coaching in the medical education continuum as having the potential to create ethical dilemmas:

1. Utility: as an employee of the university or the school of medicine, whose interests should the coach prioritize—coachee, the school, or the university? Martin Talbot points out the ethical dilemma between prioritizing the learner or the learner's eventual clients, also known as future patients.[11]

2. Autonomy: there is a slippery slope between respecting a coachee's autonomy and letting the coachee function autonomously as pointed out by Gillon.[12] The latter can be dangerous if the coachee is a medical learner participating in patient care who is found to be negligent, unprofessional, or mentally unfit. At what point should the coach keep the coachee from committing a mistake?

3. Confidentiality: in what instances can the coach break confidentiality? What if the learner is unsafe to self, and in turn, to their patients? What if the learner confides in the coach that they suffer from substance abuse? Does the coach now have the moral obligation to breach confidentiality?

4. Avoiding harm: a coach should know their limitations and know when to recommend the learner to a career mentor or academic adviser. A coach can act in the best interest of the coachee. Coaches can't serve in a position of an evaluator because a negative relationship can adversely affect the student's academic record, reduce trust, and cause harm.

5/6. Truth/justice: Shapira-Lishchinsky[13] discusses how truth and justice are intimately related in the dilemma of distributive justice against school standards in which the coach has to weigh their personal truth against the rules set by the parent organization. When these two truths differ, dissonance can arise as to which truth to abide by. The ultimate outcome for the

Vignette 2

Paula is a first-year medical student. You are meeting with her for her required spring semester coaching session. She has done very well on her exams thus far and reports adapting well to medical school. She expresses a strong interest in wanting to go into a surgical subspecialty, possibly ophthalmology or orthopedic surgery. You inquire what extracurricular activities she is involved in, and she replies that she is not participating in any outside activities so that she can focus on her grades as she knows she has to have great grades to be competitive for the specialties in which she is interested. You also inquire what she is planning to do during the summer months between year 1 and year 2. She replies that she plans to work full-time at a long-term care facility, as she is trying to minimize her educational debt. She also shares that she has been working part-time as a nurse's aide during year 1. Lastly, you inquire if she has spoken with any faculty in the fields in which she is interested, and she replies that she has not.

Thought Questions

1. What additional information would be helpful for you to know about Paula?
2. What approach might you take to assist Paula in becoming more informed about her stated specialty interests?
3. What student services personnel might be of benefit to Paula?

coachee then straddles between just and unjust based on the view of the beholder.

7. Respecting the rights of others: this fundamental principle dictates that all humans have basic rights. Specifically, addressing the hierarchy in medical education, a medical student has the same rights as a tenured professor. A grievance by either party can be problematic for a coach—whether to respect the rights of the coachee or a colleague. In these instances, the university must have a due process to ensure that everyone's rights are protected.

ADDRESSING ETHICAL DILEMMAS

Passmore et al. suggest that ethical decision-making frameworks can help coaches make informed ethical decisions. They propose a model comprising six stages: awareness; classify; time for reflection, support, and advice; initiate; option evaluation; and novate (ACTION) (Table 8.1),

TABLE 8.1 ACTION—Six Stages of Ethical Decision-Making

Awareness	Be aware of ethical codes, values, and beliefs.
Classify	Be able to classify an issue as a dilemma.
Time	Take time to reflect on the situation; seek additional support or advice if needed.
Initiate	Explore potential solutions.
Option	Weigh the different options.
Novate	Learn from the different experiences.

Adapted from The ACTION model for ethical decision-making in coaching: Passmore J. Coaching ethics: Making ethical decisions—novices and experts. *The Coaching Psychologist.* 2009;5(1):6–10.

indicating coaches should be aware of ethical codes, be able to classify an issue as a dilemma, take time to reflect, build a solution, weigh the different options, and learn from the experience.[10] This is separately confirmed by Carroll's[14] and Pryor's[15] work as early as 1998 and 1989, respectively.

Faculty development programs should discuss how to address ethical dilemmas arising in coaching relationships. Passmore suggests employing trained supervisors who can share their experience to supplement coaching competencies and help a novice coach work through real dilemmas.[9] Such supervision also has the added benefit of enhancing the ethical behavior of coaches.[1] Additionally, coaching programs should support regular meetings of the entire cohort of coaches in which members can share ethical situations in de-identified ways and process experiences together to support consistency in approach.

A coaching contract or written agreement between a coach and a coachee can provide a structural understanding and help mitigate the development of ethical dilemmas by making it easy to set boundaries; for example, the coach should be explicit about when it is appropriate to refer the coachee to a necessary support[16] service, such as an academic counselor or lead adviser for academic issues, to a physician for matters concerning physical health, and to mental health specialists for psychiatric concerns. This contract can also serve to lay down ground rules and instances when it would be permissible for the coach to breach confidentiality, such as to prevent harm to the coachee or to others. Principles of the coaching relationship by Moore et al. serve as an excellent template to start from when considering formulating a coaching agreement.[16]

Considering the existence of power differential and the reality of different lived experiences and privileges between coach and coachee, the code of ethics and ethical conduct are the anchors that provide a nonjudgmental inclusive environment for coaching to take place and foster the progress of all learners.

COACHING AND CONSIDERATIONS OF DIVERSITY, EQUITY, AND INCLUSION

Coaching is about bringing out intrinsic human resourcefulness. The coach has to truly believe in the resourcefulness of the learner and not resort to advising. The coach must enter the relationship in a state of "not knowing" to provide space and time to the coachee for self-discovery. The first step in that direction is establishing trust, which is perhaps one of the most enduring tasks of the coach. It is imperative for the coach to provide a safe environment that allows each learner to be who they are without any inhibition. The coach demonstrates respect for the coachee's perceptions, learning style, and personal being. There is unconditional acceptance of the coachee, which comes from being genuinely curious and having an open mind. Some traps that can hinder the establishment of such a trusting relationship include the coach believing they have all the answers; having judgment about some preconceived aspect of the learner, especially when the coach and coachee are from different backgrounds; imposing values on the coachee; explaining compulsively; needing to be liked; and desiring to reform the coachee. Other traps include preoccupation, unawareness, or a lack of preparation on the part of the coach.[17] Bias can get in the way of objectivity and therefore being aware of one's position, and the existence of one's own bias is critical. This may require a coach to lean into a zone of discomfort, reexamining their own beliefs and not letting prejudice get in the way.

Issues of Equity

Just as physicians have come to understand how social determinants of health drive inequities in health outcomes, coaches must recognize that educational inequities also exist and must be addressed for all health professional learners to thrive. In the context of coaching, coaches must consider the differences between equity and equality.

As defined by the *Merriam-Webster Dictionary*:
Equity: fairness or justice in the way people are treated.
Equality: the quality or state of being equal.

Specifically, in pursuit of providing equality in coaching, a coach may play an important role in identifying and potentially assisting learners in mitigating educational inequities. Failing to address inequities can result in a

Vignette 3

Dr. Pennywell, an associate professor in the department of pediatrics, has recently started coaching students to help them attain academic success. She is sitting with Harry, a first-generation rural student from a family of farmers, who is in the third year of his medical studies. Despite meeting for the fourth time since the beginning of the semester, Professor Pennywell has not been able to break the ice and is struggling to understand how to help Harry. Even though Harry is doing well in academics, Professor Pennywell finds out from colleagues that he does not seem to thrive in teams and is sometimes uncomfortable speaking with several of his classmates. She has been trying to get him to open up but instead feels that he is somewhat subtly antagonistic and disrespectful toward her; she gets frustrated, uncomfortable, and even angry. She feels guilty that the coaching conversation is not progressing and that both of them may be wasting their time.

Thought Questions

1. What could be the next step for Professor Pennywell to take care of herself?
2. How can she redirect the conversation such that Harry benefits from coaching?
3. Is this the right time to seek additional help from other colleagues/coaches/counselors about how she feels during her conversations with Harry?

fundamentally different, and therefore potentially unequal, coaching experience for learners.

Structural competency refers to a physician's ability to recognize upstream drivers of social determinants of health, such "as health care and food delivery systems, zoning laws, urban and rural infrastructures, medicalization, or even about the very definitions of illness and health."[18] Coaches should apply the same structural approach to understanding educational inequities by practicing the five core competencies as discussed in Chapter 3. Depending on their lived experiences, many learners may suffer inequities in the medical learning environment. Learners from groups underrepresented in medicine (those racial and ethnic populations that are underrepresented in the medical profession relative to their numbers in the general population),[19] those from low-income backgrounds, first-generation college educated, those who identify as LGBTQ+, those with disabilities, and others may be vulnerable to a variety of barriers and challenges. Coaches must recognize

that any struggles such learners encounter are not anchored in personal attributes but derive from unjust structural drivers that have affected prior development and ongoing experiences.

Prior to medical school, such learners from historically marginalized groups may not have had access to advisers, mentors, or family members who are well-versed in common and needed professional advancement strategies and experiences. This lack of access to resources or familiarity with needed activities for professional success can continue to exist even in medical school and residency. The "hidden" or "underground" curriculum in medical school and residency is widely recognized among learners. Even in academic courses where assessment measures are well-defined and detailed in syllabi, researchers have identified disparities in grading outcomes that have cascading impacts on career opportunities.[20] Cocurricular activities and other experiences (e.g., research, leadership, service activities, etc.) that are influential and consequential for residency selection or securing fellowship and employment opportunities may not be well known by all learners. This is particularly true for learners who do not independently establish relationships with key faculty and administrators. A coaching program adherent to ethical themes (e.g., truth, justice, respecting the rights of others) can serve as a critical bridge to ensure equal access and, therefore, promote equity for all learners.

Inequities for learners can present in many forms and develop at various times. Limited financial resources, family responsibilities, disabilities, racial inequalities, etc., are common stressors and potential sources or causes of inequity for learners. Participation in research, leadership, and service activities, as well as networking activities (e.g., specialty interest groups, professional societies, etc.) play important roles in establishing competitiveness for awards, scholarships, honor society induction, and acceptance into a residency or in achieving a fellowship or employment position. These cocurricular activities provide an avenue for a learner to develop professional relationships with faculty members in their area of interest and who, in time, may serve as mentors and provide professional references. Importantly, these contacts and experiences often play a critical role in the learner's professional identity formation and help combat imposter syndrome. Some learners lack social capital—the networks of relationships among people who live and work in a particular society, enabling that society to function effectively—to pursue and feel confident engaging in such interactions. In the course of a coaching relationship, it is imperative a coach does not make assumptions regarding a coachee's understanding of advancement within medical school and residency. Early in the coach-coachee relationship, the coach needs to assess the coachee's understanding of supplemental, extracurricular, and cocurricular activities as important components in advancing both short-term and long-term professional opportunities.

Inequities may not be fully identified until a trusting relationship has developed with the coach, and a strong ethical foundation is key to building this trust. Furthermore, general trust issues regarding institutional resources and the field of medicine overall may influence the understanding and acceptance of the coach's role and importance of coaching in professional development and career advancement among some coachees, particularly those underrepresented in medicine (UiM). Historical inequities embedded within medical education materials (e.g., visual representation of dermatologic conditions, race-based examples of diseases and conditions, etc.) and in clinical practices (e.g., historical race-based adjustments in calculating estimated glomerular filtration rate [eGFR]) can also impair a sense of inclusion. Considering that some UiM coachees may engage in a coaching relationship in a more measured, cautious fashion than their non-UiM peers, it becomes all the more important for a coach to build that trust to unearth inequities.[21]

Asking a coachee about their educational and work history can provide useful contextual information regarding professional experiences prior to and early on in medical training. Additional inquiry can also assist in a thorough understanding of potential contributors to inequity arising from past or ongoing personal conditions or situations. Challenges may exist both within the learning environment or in a coachee's personal life and relationships. When indicated, coaches can make appropriate referrals, such as to academic support and medical and psychological services. A coach is also appropriately placed to help the coachee identify potential future challenges.

With respect to career exploration and personal development, the coach does not tell the coachee what to do or whom to contact, but rather discusses, for example, how to explore and engage a faculty member for a potential opportunity. Drawing on a coachee's prior successful pursuits and experiences can provide reinforcement in their pursuit of cocurricular activities and other opportunities. Through identification of needs, contextual guidance, and avoidance of assumptions, a coach can assist a learner in developing and achieving through their own means goals they might not otherwise establish and ultimately be able to accomplish.

Understanding Challenges of Diversity and Inclusion

In the coaching relationship, because the coachee is in charge and the coach simply facilitates the process of learning and development, it is critical for the coach to step out

of the advising role. This is no small task for faculty, considering the hierarchical nature of traditional academic medicine. Coaches, therefore, would benefit significantly from understanding how lived experiences arising from socialization shape each individual, how a view of the world differs based on socialization, and how socialization may lead to biases. Understanding the science and logic behind the formation of biases (including examining one's own biases) would significantly help coaches be more effective in helping their learners.

Socialization and the Development of Bias

Socialization is the preparation of newcomers to become members of a group that already exists; the process helps individuals to think, feel, and act in ways that are appropriate for that particular group.[22] It entails the internalization of social norms, roles, and values into oneself. Society instills the ways in which individuals learn to think and behave, shaped by the context of one's circumstances, the actual content and the processes used, and the results of the contexts and processes. Socialization, therefore, begins even before we are born and is an essential component of the development of one's identity.

We are born without bias or assumptions and have no choice regarding any specific set of social identities that relate us to our ethnicity, gender, skin color, language, religion, ability status, sexual orientation, or economic class.[23] We have no initial consciousness about who we are. The characteristics of the world system include tradition, habits, stereotypes, biases, and prejudices that already exist and were built long before we existed. After birth, first or primary socialization by the people we love and trust teaches us to play the roles prescribed and abide by the existing norms and rules of society. For example, we are given a pink blanket for a girl and blue for a boy or hear phrases like "Boys don't cry," which become an automatic part of our early socialization, both intrapersonally (how we think about ourselves) and interpersonally (how we relate to others), and we do not question them. Learning during this phase is mostly observational through the formation of images of the roles and attitudes observed of the people around us.

The process of socialization continues, consciously and unconsciously, as we are exposed to messages like "Money talks" or "Girls are not good with numbers" while moving through school, places of worship, peer groups, businesses, and in particular exposure to media. This so-called secondary or adult stage involves more self-initiated role taking. A system of punishments and rewards, sanctions, and victimization keeps individuals playing by the rules as we progress through life (Fig. 8.1). Fear, ignorance, confusion, power, or powerlessness at the core of the cycle keep

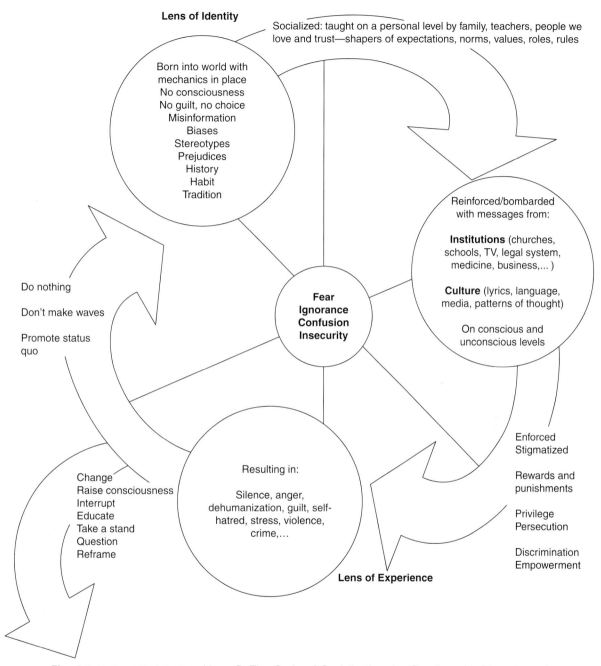

Fig. 8.1 Cycle of Socialization. Harro B. The Cycle of Socialization. In: *Readings for Diversity and Social Justice: An Anthology on Racism, Anti-Semitism, Sexism, Heterosexism, Ableism, and Classism.* New York, NY: Routledge; 2000:15–21.

the process alive. Our identities are therefore shaped by the forces of socialization encompassing perceptions and experiences felt through our cultural lens. This lens is neither universal nor objective but conforms to the collective experience of the group to which we belong.[24] For example, being a man leads to different experiences from being a woman, being rich produces something entirely different from being poor, and having a disability is different from being able-bodied, and these experiences are often hard to fathom by members of the other group.

Learning what is expected by group members takes place through a variety of mediums that are mostly non-verbal, such as watching and comparing ourselves to others, television, song lyrics, movies, and social media, and these lived experiences are very different between groups. Robin DiAngelo explains in her book *White Fragility: Why It Is So Hard for White People to Talk about Racism* that the concept of pretty has no meaning without the concept of ugly and smart means little without the idea of not smart.[24] It is important to remember that we generally fail to fully recognize the circumstances of the other groups, in particular the disadvantaged group from the position of the privileged. Knowing that lived experiences can potentially be dramatically different between a coach and a coachee, it is imperative for the coach to be cognizant of the existence of differences in order to prevent misunderstanding and potentially endangering the coaching relationship. This also argues for greater diversity among coaches to broaden the perspective of any institution's coaching cohort.

Lived experiences shape the development of unconscious bias in all of us that may hinder effective coaching unintentionally. The development of bias is linked to affiliation, a basic human survival instinct. Affiliation serves to create and preserve self-identity and helps us identify with those around us such that we are not left alone, vulnerable, and exposed.[25] A neuroimaging study in Jennifer Eberhardt's lab demonstrated that specific areas in the temporal lobe set in motion in- and out-group distinctions (us vs. them), informed by relationships with the world around us, to help us distinguish familiar from unfamiliar and friend from foe.[25] Because the conscious mind can process only a fraction of the total information that the brain can process at a given time, a lot of the processing of distinctions happens subconsciously. Without any volitional control, the brain groups similar things together in order to simplify, organize, and make sense of the overload of information. Our thoughts, attitudes, and instincts about and against people are thus formed because of associations and affiliations, skin color being one of the basic first cues for assigning group membership. The amygdala plays an important role in this grouping mechanism. It generates fear and distrust very rapidly of anything that poses a danger, such as any kind of unfamiliarity, without conscious knowledge. Socialization produces experiences, memories, and unconscious biases, which the amygdala labels and categorizes as "like me"/in-group and "not like me"/out-group. This categorization helps the brain make judgments quickly and efficiently based on heuristics or instincts and not reasoning or logic; this process is not arbitrary and is essential for our survival. Studies using functional magnetic resonance imaging (fMRI) demonstrate that different parts of the brain are used for discerning "familiar" and "unfamiliar" situations providing a biologic explanation for the difference between heuristic and formal logic. Importantly, when we are tired or stressed, we fall back on instincts, bypassing rational thinking. The phenomenon of in-group and out-group categorization hinders our understanding of people unlike us (the concept of "otherness") as it dampens the sensitivity to those who look different and therefore naturally makes us susceptible to misjudgments. Being aware of the existence of such unconscious behavior in all individuals can be beneficial in the coaching context and potentially help minimize judgmental errors and the risk of causing unintended harm.

The oversimplified generalizations about social groups without taking into account individual differences are labeled stereotypes. Stereotypes can be positive—usually of one's own group—or negative about other groups. Prejudice is prejudgment about another person based on the social group to which an individual belongs. It consists of attitudes, thoughts, and feelings, including stereotypes based on little or no actual experience about a group, such as believing elderly people are lazy. All humans have prejudices that are created based on the information gained from the society around us. The prevailing belief that prejudice is bad causes us to deny the unavoidable reality of its existence in each of us.[24] Prejudices may lead to discrimination that can take the form of ignoring, exclusion, threats, ridicule, slander of, and violence against members of other groups. Prejudice alters our instincts about people and situations. Bias often surfaces when an individual does not align with expected standards in society making us instinctively suspicious.[26] Related to affiliation, we tend to be rigid in the acceptance of the "culturally alike" and rejection of the "culturally unlike" individuals. This thinking is directly linked to the preservation of the self and the identity resulting in in-group favoritism that can be explicit (prejudice against or active denigration of an out-group) or subtle and implicit (bias in favor of the in-group). This unconscious behavior and decision-making may lead to discrediting those with a different attribute such as skin color or physical ability, resulting in discrediting the person's whole social identity. It is important for coaches to recognize that we are vulnerable to unconsciously denying the whole identity of another individual based on certain attributes that are different from ours.

In the context of coaching it is crucial to bear in mind that unconscious bias is pervasive, does not necessarily align with our declared beliefs, and is malleable because of the neuroplasticity of our brain. Implicit bias is hard to pinpoint simply because it is hidden. Among all the identity biases that exist, race and gender are two commonly encountered ones. Although there is no biologic category of race, race as a social construct has a profound significance and shapes every aspect of our lives, including survival, life expectancy, careers, opportunities, and clinical management of health conditions that may lead to errors.

It is now recognized that children as young as three may have well-defined racial preferences that are learned from the nonverbal behaviors displayed by surrounding adults, independent of their verbal behaviors, which lead children to behave prosocially toward the recipient of the positive nonverbal signals.[27,28] Thus prejudice is learned in childhood without even being aware of it. Color-blind socialization practices of not discussing race with children and ignoring children's observations about intergroup conflict show that mothers' cross-race friendship predicted their children's racial attitudes: children of White mothers with more non-White friends showed fewer racial biases than children whose White mothers had fewer non-White friends.[29] Parents use different racial socialization methods, like "cultural socialization, preparation for bias, instilling mistrust, egalitarian or colorblindness, or silence about race" according to the circumstances (urban vs. rural, higher vs. lower socioeconomic group, Black vs. White, and so on); the impact of these strategies on the identity of children and youth and life in general is important as it affects how we bring ourselves to the world.[30] Based on what has been discussed thus far, it may be surmised that biases and prejudices may show up unintentionally during any interaction; learning to recognize differences with intentionality may be hugely beneficial for coaches.

Diverse Populations in Medical Training

Acknowledging that structural drivers shape academic faculties, cohorts of coaches recruited from teaching faculty are unlikely to fully reflect the diversity of the program's coachees. Institutions should make efforts to assemble cohorts of coaches who represent various dimensions of diversity and provide group development opportunities to broaden one another's perspectives and ensure all coaches are prepared to interact with learners of varied backgrounds.

As mentioned previously, there are people from multiple groups within the medical profession who are marginalized, including first-generation college educated, those from low-income backgrounds, those who identify as LGBTQ+, those with disabilities, and others. Given the profound societal impact of structural racism, members of racial and ethnic populations UiM deserve resources to account for inequities. Structural racism refers to "a system in which public policies, institutional practices, cultural representations, and other norms work in various, often reinforcing ways to perpetuate racial group inequity. It identifies dimensions of our history and culture that have allowed privileges associated with 'whiteness' and disadvantages associated with 'color' to endure and adapt over time. Structural racism is not something that a few people or institutions choose to practice. Instead, it has been a feature of the social, economic, and political systems in which we all exist."[31]

Work is ongoing to increase diversity in medicine in order to expand career opportunities, reduce health inequities, provide culturally responsive patient and community care, improve clinical training with appropriate classroom discussions, and appropriately prepare all learners to work in multicultural settings that foster equitable access to care by any physician. A review of twenty-eight studies conducted between 1980 and 2012 to understand the experiences of UiM students in the learning environment revealed "almost unanimously that these learners experienced less supportive social and less positive learning environments, have been subjected to discrimination and racial harassment, and have been more likely to perceive that their race negatively affected their medical school experiences" compared with non-UiM students.[32] Interviews with UiM students also revealed that they had difficulty forming study groups with non-UiM students.[32] Perceptions not only influence unconscious bias that affects outcomes but also undermine performance. It is now proven through many studies that performance is impaired when individuals are concerned about conforming to a negativity bias. Supporting this view, Orom et al. found that the expectation that UiM students would fare worse in standardized tests and have higher attrition rates creates a stereotype threat that undermines performance and contributes to those assumptions becoming reality.[32] As a corollary, it can be expected that the existing climate in academic medicine may be hampering the willingness of UiM learners to choose medicine as a career despite global efforts in enhancing recruitment of learners from UiM groups. Undoubtedly the performance issues arise in part from inequities in K-12 and undergraduate education, but the opportunity exists to adjust for these discrepancies in academic medicine, especially through coaching.

Although medical schools have been proactively working on policies and processes to recruit learners from UiM backgrounds, this has not translated to universal inclusive practices and tailored coaching needs. The learning environment and coaching needs of UiM learners have been further explored in a study by Najibi et al.;[21] the authors ascertain that in contrast to students who represent the majority, UiM students would like coaches to recognize their cultural context during coaching. Coaching inherently entails vulnerability from both the coach and the coachee; Najibi's study shows that UiM students find it stressful to share vulnerability.[21] In contrast, the coaches' perceptions of the needs and expectations were not substantially different for the two different groups. This creates disharmony. Knowing that, in general, the majority of the faculty in academic medicine are not from underrepresented groups, the coaching relationship with UiM learners requires particular attention and professional development for faculty to be successful. Without appropriate training and awareness among faculty, coaching may cause unintentional harm. Learners may be unintentionally made to feel invisible, feel not included, fear discrimination, experience lower self-esteem, and have increased stress and anxiety. This unintentional harm can also include impaired performance and lead to physical and mental illness as a result of chronic stress. Bias can be further internalized and become self-fulfilling. All of these factors are observed during residency as well.

The Coach's Need for Self-awareness to Recognize and Mitigate Bias

Hinged upon the basic ethical coaching principle of "do no harm," we can draw upon gender equality expert Michelle King's 4Ps of inequity (Table 8.2)[33] to help mitigate race-related inequities that exist in medicine. The current overwhelming focus on policies and processes for recruitment of UiM belies the lived experiences of UiM and may

TABLE 8.2	Addressing Inequity
Policies	Policy for enhanced recruitment of minority students into medical school
Processes	The process to increase reach to diverse groups of students in various dimensions
Practices	How faculty interact with diverse patients; how faculty interact with diverse groups of students and residents in the classroom and in the clinics
Personal beliefs	Biases and prejudices; e.g., negative perception for availing of maternity/paternity leave

Adapted from The Four Ps of Inequity: King M. How to address gender inequity in your organization. *Harv Bus Rev.* September 16, 2020.

simply reinforce exclusivity unintentionally. More work is required to embrace practices and address personal beliefs in order to provide an appropriate coaching environment for all types of learners, especially because a coaching relationship may often entail a majority-minority pair. Even though some of the implicit biases develop as a mechanism of survival, these are not necessarily hardwired in the brain or inherited. Social psychologists suggest that bias effects can change depending on the context, and therefore it is possible to change bias in an individual, though the change may neither be easy nor achieved overnight. Faculty development is therefore critical in making the change toward being inclusive of differences in the coachee. Understanding biases at the individual (interpersonal) level make it possible to start to understand the societal and structural inequities. The most common blind spot is believing that others have it and you don't; the developmental work starts with the recognition that we all have biases and blind spots. The Implicit Association Test (IAT) helps learn about one's thoughts and feelings outside of conscious awareness.[34] The IAT test by measuring reaction time makes deductions about the strength of associations between concepts and evaluations of stereotypes. As an example, whether White and Black are equally associated with human words and animal words tests the dehumanizing of Black people by White people.[34] It is important to recognize that IAT reaction time may not necessarily be related to implicit bias and does not necessarily predict behavior. It may be just one way to illuminate an individual's mental workings.

Implicit bias is layered and complicated. Therefore unconscious bias training is complex, outcomes are hard to measure, and evidence of effectiveness in reducing bias is lacking.[24] Ironically, unconscious bias training may normalize bias. What is often found useful and highly recommended for faculty development is reflecting on one's identity to fully recognize the privileges or lack thereof in one's life and bringing to the surface how one became aware of one's identity(ies), through critical incidents (Fig. 8.2). Being aware of one's identity helps explore how it shaped one's experiences and view of the world and how it is expressed in life. These narratives are neither unique nor objective but belong to the collective message received as members of a larger shared culture or group.[24] The reflections are essentially meant to help us know ourselves better such that we are more open and mindful about receiving other's life experiences and are able to minimize the impact as educators and caregivers. Lindsey and colleagues have used reflection-based diversity training that "encourages participants to think about their past experiences regarding prejudice, review what happened, how they responded, what they wished they would have done differently in the situation, and what they hope to do differently in the

---

Self-identities

We are very attached to our stories, our identities of who we are. But how do we know what those are and how we developed those identities? Weave a story on your belief, of your identity.

I am "_____" (a White woman, an Indian man, a Black surgeon, a French Moroccan singer, middle-aged male physician, middle-aged woman, an Asian engineer . .). Whatever identity you align with, fill in the blanks. Think of the most important identity (at the most two) you consider about yourself.

Reflect on the following questions as appropriate (10 minutes)

- **When** did you first learn that there was something called gender (if being a woman or man is the strongest identity), or race (if race is your strongest identity), ethnicity, or XXXXX (your strongest identity)?
- **How** did you learn about this identity of yours? Was it from a family member? Was it through a joke by a friend?
- **What** was that experience/incident? These are called **critical incidents** that shape who we are and what we think of other people.

Recollect that story in your mind (5 minutes).

The objectives are

- to bring honor and awareness to our identity; shine a light on what we carry that may be influencing how we make choices.
- to reflect on
  - How has this identity shaped my experiences in life?
  - Are we sending signals from identity without our awareness (our blind self)?
  - How are these signals affecting the way we show up and/or interact with colleagues and/or direct reports who are simply different from us?

Fig. 8.2 Reflection on Identity.

---

future."[35] They found that those who benefit from this training are those with high internal motivation to reduce prejudice; in the context of academic coaching, this method of training can be particularly relevant considering that all faculty who engage in coaching do so with the sole purpose of helping learners; are very likely to have a high motivation to succeed; and therefore, as a corollary, want to reduce their own prejudice.

There is an inherent inertia in staying silent about diversity, in particular regarding racism, which does not frequently get discussed or taught in educational settings. Discussing race openly and honestly makes some individuals go silent, can bring up arguments, makes some people defensive, and if not handled well can prevent productive discussion and knowledge about race while holding the racial hierarchy in place.[24] A commonly used approach to dealing with racial differences is to stay color-blind and not "see" race in an effort to endorse meritocracy; this ideology is based on the fact that "recognizing race is a precondition to racism, and thus failing to recognize race reduces racism."[29] However, being color-blind invalidates the lived experiences of others. Because of a lack of conversation and learning about race, many hold a simplistic understanding of racism in today's context. Some think of this as binary—that being racist means intentionally disliking others because of their race and therefore being immoral, whereas not being racist equals good. In reality, understanding racism is about exploring structural drivers of the racial socialization and racial dynamics that exist in society.[24] It is worth remembering that race was developed as a tool to divide and control populations during European colonization; there is nothing biologic as race, which is simply a phenotype.[36] Over time, the meaning of race has shifted to suit political needs and to assert inferiority over darker-skinned populations.[36] This assertion has led to significant health advantages to White people in comparison with other groups.[37] An example resource to support discussions exploring racial socialization and developing understanding of the existence of racial dynamics and their influence on people on both sides of the divide is the reading guide accompanying *White Fragility.*[24] A potential tool to support the necessary personal work and reflection in understanding how racism exists today and surfaces in our daily interactions is the workbook *Me and White Supremacy: Combat Racism, Change the World, and Become a Good Ancestor* by Layla Saad, whose work derives from her passion to be a good ancestor to subsequent generations.[38] Author Rhonda Magee proposes approaching the difficult situations of racism that may arrive in daily life from the perspective of mindfulness.[39] In a similar vein, Michael Mensah proposes that acknowledging White privilege is the first step in the payment of "majority taxes," which has the intention of changing practices related to race in academic medicine.[40] All of these considerations should be part of the ongoing development work for a coach who wishes to work with medical learners from marginalized groups.

Techniques to Support Inclusive Coaching

Debiasing is a lifelong self-developmental process. A conscious effort in taking the time to make decisions, instead of using heuristics to decide, helps de-automatize decision-making, which in coaching may mean not drawing conclusions about coachees and instead taking the time to understand their life circumstances. A conscious effort in avoiding categorizations and generalizations and instead focusing on individual differences while speaking (e.g., instead of saying "boys like dinosaurs," one may say "this boy likes dinosaurs") are helpful strategies that avoid stereotypical ideation. Microaggressions can be committed by either the coach or coachee. Microaggressions are "brief and commonplace daily verbal, behavioral, or environmental indignities, whether intentional or unintentional, that communicate hostile, derogatory, or negative slights and insults toward marginalized groups."[41] It is important to address the microaggression and not the aggressor. Suggested strategies include willingness to accept when bias is pointed out by focusing on the message and not the messenger, wanting to learn about others' experiences, and being comfortable with differences. Coaches may invite coachees to provide real-time reflections on inclusivity.

Perspective taking, which involves a conscious attempt to visualize and feel another person's viewpoint, can be particularly effective in reducing implicit bias.[26] To understand this formally in a study, researchers showed nurses pictures of either Black or White patients with expressions of pain and asked how much pain medication they would recommend. When told to use their best judgment, significantly more pain medication was recommended to White than Black patients whereas when instructed to imagine how the patient felt, the recommendations were equal regardless of race.[26]

Although perspective taking and paying attention to the body language and attitude of the learner can be beneficial in understanding the circumstances of the student or resident, these can also lead to misunderstanding and misinterpretation. As Nicholas Epley suggests, based on his research on mind reading, it is better to ask questions that reveal the circumstances and therefore enable true growth for the learner rather than striving to put oneself in another's shoes.[42] In coaching parlance this is referred to as powerful questioning that moves away from the "why" and instead embraces "what" and "how" questions.

It is imperative for coaches to listen with full attention to all the facts learners provide along with their feelings without having an internal agenda to see certain outcomes; this type of listening is called level 3 listening[43] and can be learned with practice. Author and professor Richard Boyatzis, one of the leading experts in the field of leadership development, emotional intelligence, and behavioral change, promulgates neuroscience-based coaching with compassion in precipitating change and growth in the coachee.[44] Continuing along the lines of compassionate coaching, we may bring to mind nonviolent communication, which espouses connecting with our own selves and with others in a manner that allows giving and receiving information compassionately. Thus, when the coachee expresses candidly and the coach receives empathetically, communication becomes authentic. The coach observes the actions of the learner, is able to understand the feelings behind the actions, and senses the need behind those actions; with this knowledge, the coach can effectively facilitate the process of powerful questioning leading to growth and development of the students and residents.[45] In this environment there is full trust; real rapport is established; and the coach and coachee mirror each other in gestures, language, body posture, pace, and energy; the mirror neuron system in the brain that imitates actions done by and emotions of others become fully engaged.[46]

Motivational interviewing (MI) and appreciative inquiry (AI) are two other questioning techniques that have been successfully applied to coaching. Coaches often struggle to overcome resistance to change in coachees. MI can be useful in such situations because motivational interviewing is facilitative and collaborative rather than prescriptive. It is goal oriented instead of person focused. Importantly, MI endeavors to speak to internal motivation, as opposed to external, and therefore has the potential for a long-lasting effect. The MI process starts with an assessment of the coachee's readiness for change and then moves to designing plans that cater to the individual needs of the learner, leading to a firm commitment to change. Coaches are expected to be skillful in reflective listening and to be empathetic.[47] If conducted appropriately, a coaching session using MI methodology may appear like a well-synchronized dance between the coach and the coachee.

AI, as discussed in Chapter 1, is a positive, strengths-based methodology to learning and development and can be extremely beneficial in building confidence. AI is based on finding the positive stories in life that can help build the preferred future the coachee envisions.[48]

CONCLUSION

Coaching is a powerful method for developing self-directed lifelong learning. However, for a coaching program to be successful in academic medicine, which has a legacy of marginalization and structural racism, it is important to be thoughtful in designing appropriate faculty development based on ethics and inclusion. This development should be an ongoing endeavor and not a one-time activity. The benefit to learners from a well-trained coach can be transformative, especially for coachees from marginalized groups. For faculty, the personal and professional development associated with such investment can be highly rewarding.

TAKE-HOME POINTS

1. Coaches can lean on an abundance of available ethical principles but should know that these alone will not sustain a coaching relationship. Ethical dilemmas will inevitably arise and require self-awareness, reflection, and willingness to seek help.
2. A coach can provide triage, routing the coachee to the appropriate referral, making sure all learners have appropriate resources to be successful regardless of personal or social circumstances.
3. Coaches have to be aware that the road traveled by the coachee is unique and should strive to appreciate each coachee's starting point and journey.
4. When addressing diversity in a coaching relationship, the coach must avoid making assumptions and rely instead on thoughtful inquiry. Making a coachee feel included has its roots in these initial encounters.
5. The importance of the coach's inner work in terms of understanding one's own biases, habits, and preferences through self-organization of body, mind, and heart cannot be underestimated; it is this inner work that allows the coach to keep an open mind and successfully engage the learner.

QUESTIONS FOR FURTHER THOUGHT

1. What resources do coaches have to preserve their relationship with coachees when confronted with ethical dilemmas, and how can these resources be made available to coaches?
2. What systems should medical schools and residency programs have in place to assess and address the varying educational needs of marginalized populations?
3. How can coaches learn to appreciate the unique learning environment of a coachee from a marginalized population and pay particular attention to cultural contexts so as to not unintentionally cause more harm, including attrition?

ANNOTATED BIBLIOGRAPHY

DiAngelo R. *White fragility: Why It's So Hard for White People to Talk About Racism* (Audiobook Narrated by Amy Landon). Beacon Press; 2018.
  A well-written narrative that is likely to capture the attention of anyone wanting to dive deeper to understand why color blindness is not possible and how to learn to cope with racism.
Harro B. The Cycle of Socialization. *Readings for Diversity and Social Justice: An Anthology on Racism, Sexism and Semitism, heterosexism, classism, and ableism.* New York, NY: Routledge. 2000:15–21.
  This provides a very clear picture of how socialization is responsible for the view we hold of the world, often without our conscious awareness. Anyone wanting to know more about the development of unconscious bias is likely to benefit from Harro's article.
Implicit Association Test. Project Implicit. https://implicit.harvard.edu/implicit/takeatest.html. Accessed July 30, 2021.
  A great resource to start to understand unconscious bias one may be carrying.

International Coaching Federation Global Board of Directors. International Coaching Federation. ICF Code of Ethics. https://coachfederation.org/code-of-ethics. Adopted September 2019. Accessed July 30, 2021.

This serves as a comprehensive list of ethical standards to abide by in a coaching relationship.

Passmore J, Mortimer L. Ethics in coaching. In Boyce LA, Hernez-Broome G, Kraut AI, eds. *Advancing Executive Coaching: Setting the Course for Successful Leadership Coaching.* San Francisco, CA: Jossey-Bass; 2011:205–227.

This article is a great discussion of ethical principles, how they naturally lend themselves to dilemmas, and how a coach can rely on ethical decision-making frameworks to make more informed ethical decisions.

Saad LF. *Me and White Supremacy: Combat Racism, Change the World, and Become a Good Ancestor.* Naperville, IL: Sourcebooks; 2020.

An excellent resource for anyone wanting to look at one's unconscious thinking about racism and to address one's blind spots. Though it is focused on race, the principles may be applied to any privileged situation. Any coach would benefit from working through this workbook as it will help one deal with diverse groups of learners.

REFERENCES

1. Ramanathan R. Ethics in Coaching. Coacharya. https://coacharya.com/blog/ethics-in-coaching/. Published January 2, 2020. Accessed July 30, 2021.
2. International Coaching Federation Global Board of Directors. International Coaching Federation. International Coaching Federation Code of Ethics. https://coachfederation.org/code-of-ethics. Adopted September 2019. Accessed July 30, 2021.
3. International Association of Coaching. Ethical principles. https://certifiedcoach.org/about/ethics/. Published 2019. Accessed July 30, 2021.
4. Association for Coaching. The Global Code of Ethics for Coaches, Mentors and Supervisors. https://www.associationforcoaching.com/page/AboutCodeEthics. Updated May 1, 2018. Accessed July 30, 2021.
5. International Coaching Community. ICC Standards and Code of Ethics. https://internationalcoachingcommunity.com/standards-and-ethics/. Published 2020. Accessed July 30, 2021.
6. American Psychological Association. Ethical Principles of Psychologists and Code of conduct. https://www.apa.org/ethics/code. Accessed July 30, 2021.
7. Institute of Coaching. Coaching competencies. https://www.instituteofcoaching.org/resources/coaching-competencies. Accessed July 30, 2021.
8. Brennan D, Wildflower L. Ethics in Coaching. In: Cox E, Bachkirova T, Clutterbuck D, eds. *The Complete Handbook of Coaching.* 2nd ed. London: Sage Publications; 2018:431–432.
9. Passmore J. Coaching ethics: Making ethical decisions–novices and experts. *The Coaching Psychologist.* 2009;5(1):6–10.
10. Passmore J, Mortimer L. Ethics in coaching. In: Boyce LA, Hernez-Broome G, Kraut AI, eds. *Advancing Executive Coaching: Setting the Course for Successful Leadership Coaching.* San Francisco, CA: Jossey-Bass; 2011:205–227.
11. Talbot M. Ethical issues in guidance and counselling in medical education: conflicts in a learner-centered approach and a hermeneutic resolution. *Br J Guid Counc.* 2000;28(1):125–134.
12. Gillon R. Autonomy and the principle of respect for autonomy*Philosophical Medical Ethics.* Chichester, England: Wiley; 1986:60.
13. Shapira-Lishchinsky O. Teachers' critical incidents: Ethical dilemmas in teaching practice. *Teach Educ.* 2011;27(3):648–656.
14. Carroll M. Ethical issues in workplace counselling. In: Crawford M, Edwards R, Kydd L, eds. *Taking Issue: Debates in Counselling and Guidance in Education.* London: Open University Press; 1998:19.
15. Pryor RGL. Conflicting responsibilities: a case study of an ethical dilemma for psychologists working in organisations. *Aust Psychol.* 1989;24(2):293–305.
16. Moore M, Jackson E, Tschannen-Moran B. Design Thinking. In: Moore M, Jackson E, Tschannen-Moran B, eds. *Coaching Psychology Manual.* 2nd ed. Philadelphia, PA: Wolters Kluwer; 2016:125–140.
17. Rogers J. *Coaching Skills: A Handbook.* 3rd ed.: Open University Press McGraw Hill; 2012 Chapter 3.
18. Metzl JM, Hansen H. Structural competency: theorizing a new medical engagement with stigma and inequality. *Soc Sci Med.* 2014;103:126–133.
19. Underrepresented in Medicine Definition. Association of American Medical Colleges. https://www.aamc.org/what-we-do/diversity-inclusion/underrepresented-in-medicine. Accessed January 5, 2022.
20. Hauer KE, Lucey CR. Core Clerkship Grading: The Illusion of Objectivity. *Acad Med.* 2019 Apr;94(4):469–472.
21. Najibi S, Carney PA, Thayer EK, Deiorio NM. Differences in Coaching Needs Among Underrepresented Minority Medical Students. *Fam Med.* 2019;51(6):516–522.
22. Persell CH. Becoming a Member of Society Through Socialization*Understanding Society: An Introduction to Sociology.* 3rd ed. New York, NY: Harper & Row, Publishers, Inc; 1990:98–107.
23. Harro B. *The Cycle of Socialization. Readings for Diversity and Social Justice: An Anthology on Racism, Sexism and Semitism, Heterosexism,Classism, and Ableism.* New York, NY: Routledge; 2000:15–21.
24. DiAngelo R. *White Fragility: Why It's So Hard for White People to Talk About Racism (Audiobook Narrated by Amy Landon).* Boston: Beacon Press; 2018.
25. Eberhardt JL. *Biased: Uncovering the Hidden Prejudice That Shapes What We See, Think, and Do.* London: Penguin Books; 2019.
26. Agarwal P. *Sway: Unravelling Unconscious Bias.* London: Bloomsbury Sigma; 2020.
27. Castelli L, Nesdale D. Learning social attitudes: children's sensitivity to the nonverbal behaviors of adult models

during interracial interactions. *Pers Soc Psychol Bull.* 2008;34(11):1504–1513.

28. Skinner AL, Meltzoff AN, Olson KR. Catching" social bias: exposure to biased nonverbal signals creates social biases in preschool children. *Psychol Sci.* 2017;28(2):216–224.

29. Pahlke E, Bigler RS, Suizzo M-A. Relations between color-blind socialization and children's racial bias: evidence from European American mothers and their preschool children. *Child Dev.* 2012;83(4):1164–1179.

30. Csizmadia A. Racial Socialization in the United States. In: Shehan CL, ed. *The Wiley Blackwell Encyclopedia of Family Studies.* Hoboken, NJ: John Wiley & Sons, Ltd; 2016.

31. Glossary for Understanding the Dismantling Structural Racism/Promoting Racial Equity Analysis. The Aspen Institute. https://www.aspeninstitute.org/wp-content/uploads/files/content/docs/rcc/RCC-Structural-Racism-Glossary.pdf. Accessed July 30, 2021.

32. Orom H, Semalulu T, Underwood W. The social and learning environments experienced by underrepresented minority medical students: a narrative review. *Acad Med.* 2013;88:1765–1777.

33. King M. How to address gender inequity in your organization. *Harv Bus Rev.* September 16, 2020.

34. Implicit Association Test. Project Implicit. https://implicit.harvard.edu/implicit/takeatest.html. Accessed July 30, 2021.

35. Lindsey A, King E, Amber B, Sabat I, Ahmad A. Examining why and for whom reflection diversity training works. *Personnel Assessment and Decisions.* 2019;5(2):82–89.

36. Cerdena JP, Plaisime MV, Tsai J. From race-based to race-conscious medicine: how anti-racist uprisings call us to act. *Lancet.* 2020;396:1125–1128.

37. Jones CP, Truman BI, Elam-Evans LD, Jones CA, Jones CY, Jiles R, Rumisha SF, Perry GS. Using "socially assigned race" to probe white advantages in health status. *Eth Dis.* 2008;18:496–504.

38. Saad LF. *Me and White Supremacy: Combat Racism, Change the World, and Become a Good Ancestor.* Naperville, IL: Sourcebooks; 2020.

39. Magee RV. *The Inner Work of Racial Justice: Healing Ourselves and Transforming Our Communities Through Mindfulness.* New York: Tarcher Perigee (Penguin Random House LLC); 2019.

40. Mensah MO. Majority Taxes - Toward Antiracist Allyship in Medicine. *N Engl J Med.* July 23, 2020;383(4): e23(1)–e23(2).

41. Sue DW. Racial microaggressions in everyday life. *American Psychologist.* 2007;62:271–286.

42. Epley N. *Mindwise: How We Understand What Others Think, Believe, Feel and Want.* New York: Alfred Knopf; 2014 Chapter 8.

43. Kimsey-House H, Kimsey-House K, Sandahl P, Whitworth L. *Co-Active Coaching: Changing Business, Transforming Lives.* 3rd edition Boston, MA: Nicholas Brealey Publishing; 2011. Chapter 3.

44. nSmith M, Boyatzis RE, Van Oosten E. Coach with compassion. *Leadership Excellence.* 2012;29(3):10.

45. Rosenberg M. Nonviolent Communication, A Language of Life. 3rd edition. Encinitas: PuddleDancer Press; 2015 Chapter 1.

46. Rizzolatti G. The mirror neuron system and its function in humans. *Anat Embryol.* 2005;210:419–421.

47. Passmore J. Addressing deficit performance through coaching—using motivational interviewing for performance improvement at work. *Int Coach Psychol Rev.* 2007;2(3):265–274.

48. Gordon S. Appreciative inquiry coaching. *Int Coach Psych Rev.* 2008;3(1):19–31.

9

Examples of Successful Coaching Programs

Hilit F. Mechaber, Donna Elliott, Micaela Godzich, Antwione Haywood, and Jennifer R. Miller

LEARNING OBJECTIVES

1. Describe both undergraduate and graduate medical education models of an academic coaching program for personal and professional development.
2. Identify key elements to consider when designing an academic coaching program.
3. Identify barriers that may be encountered when implementing novel programs.
4. Recognize the need to engage stakeholders, define resources, and identify appropriate time needed to plan a successful program.

CHAPTER OUTLINE

CHAPTER SUMMARY

In this chapter, we review the different opportunities for coaching in medical education and provide examples of coaching programs in undergraduate and graduate medical education as well as an example of a peer-to-peer model. These examples serve as templates for institutions considering implementation of an academic coaching program and offer insight into the various dimensions to consider while planning. We identify resources needed to successfully support programs, review key stakeholders, and describe logistics required to implement and assess these novel programs.

INTRODUCTION

How can medical schools best welcome and prepare newly arrived students in ways that are inclusive and appropriate? How can residency programs build community through coaching? How can medicine adapt when there is a global pandemic that requires learners and teachers to learn and connect in unfamiliar ways? Coaching is a secret ingredient of student success, and it can help answer these questions. At its core, we place value in the student tapping into intrinsic motivators, reflective practice, and critical thinking. The beauty of coaching is that we can inspire students to remember they are the experts and the leaders in their own lives. The coaches provide their coachees with the time and the safe space to reflect upon themselves and respond to skillfully posed questions. These powerful questions nudge students to discover how they can transport themselves from where they are and who they are to where they want to be and who they want to become. The practice of generous listening without offering advice results in enhanced levels of not only perspective taking, but self-compassion. Coaching puts the coachee in the driver's seat to develop resiliency or, in other words, the ability to remain nimble in the face of challenge. Cultivating resilience is important as an antidote to burnout. Individual factors of resilience include the capacity for self-monitoring, setting limits, and attitudes that promote constructive engagement with the difficult challenges. The following models are examples of effective coaching programs.

MODEL 1: UNDERGRADUATE MEDICAL EDUCATION PROFESSIONAL DEVELOPMENT COACHING PROGRAM

Donna Elliott

Description of the Program

At our medical school, the University of Southern California Keck School of Medicine, we created a professional development coaching program for medical students to facilitate them reaching their full potential as both medical students and student physicians. The program supports the development of an open connection between coach and coachee and fosters a longitudinal, open relationship throughout medical school that includes required meetings and the opportunity to connect for additional conversations as needed. The role of a coach is to provide an emotionally safe, nonjudgmental, and unconditionally supportive atmosphere for the student and demonstrate vulnerability by sharing relevant professional and personal experiences, as appropriate, to build a trusting relationship. A coach may also occasionally mentor or advise as it is extremely difficult to fully and distinctly separate these roles.

At matriculation students are randomly assigned to faculty coaches. The coach-coachee pairs meet during orientation week to begin introductions, opening the lines of communication and beginning to build trust. Students and coaches review and sign a coaching contract at an early meeting. The contract defines the relationship and expectations for both the coach and student. Coaches receive ongoing, comprehensive data about student performance that include student narrative evaluations, test scores, grades, absence requests, professionalism lapses, peer evaluations, evaluation completion rates, and other surveys or relevant assignments. Prior to each meeting, using a dashboard designed specifically for this purpose, coaches review data and submitted materials and identify areas for discussion with the student. The coaches assist in identifying SMART goals (specific, measurable, achievable, relevant, time-based) and in creating a plan to achieve them. Coaching sessions are documented to provide a record for the student and coach to refer to in future meetings to assess and promote professional growth and development. During subsequent meetings the coach and student will review progress toward those goals and make any needed course corrections. This documentation is only available to coaches, students, and the assistant dean of student affairs, who serves as the director of the coaching program.

Coaches are expected to use the resources of the medical school for referrals and support and are not expected to resolve all issues. The coaches work closely with the office of medical student wellness, the office of academic support services, and the office of student affairs to ensure all concerns are addressed and all students receive appropriate support. This process is monitored by the assistant dean for student affairs.

Program Objectives

1. Provide a safe space for reflection on academic, personal, and professional performance.
2. Ensure well-being and assist with the development of skills to develop resilience.
3. Assist in goal setting and hold students accountable to the identified goals.
4. Encourage students to establish habits of continuous reflection, goal setting, and lifelong learning.

Program Logistics

The coaching program is embedded in the Professional Identity Formation (PIF) course. This course spans the preclinical phase, which includes the first 18 months of medical school, although coaches continue to work with students for all 4 years. As is the case in other coaching programs, coaches may serve multiple roles. The coaches work with a partner coach, and together they serve as faculty facilitators for 24 students. The coachees for both coaches are the students in each cohort of incoming medical students. The PIF course provides the framework for the coaching model and affords students the opportunity to gain knowledge and build skills to facilitate personal and professional growth.

Each coach follows a group of students for all 4 years, with more frequent meetings for students in the preclinical phase. Coaches meet with each student approximately five times in the preclinical phase at designated times and then continue with approximately one scheduled meeting per semester until graduation. At each coaching session general issues are reviewed, including academic performance and professionalism. Included topics are relevant to the specific developmental milestones critical to medical school. Mandatory assignments that were preassigned are reviewed during the meetings. Additional agenda items can be added at the request of the student. Each coach will have 12 students from each class and no more than 24 students total; student groups will be members of alternating classes.

Coaches are clinical faculty at the medical school and are available to students between meetings as needed. Students will not be assigned to or be evaluated by their coach or noncoach PIF instructor during clinical rotations. Interested faculty must apply to be a coach and agree to the requirements of the program if selected. The application and selection process is rigorous, and the assistant dean for student affairs and the codirector of the PIF course conduct the recruitment and make the final selections. The coaches come from a variety of specialties, including primary care and surgical subspecialties. The time commitment for each coach is one half day per week, and they are funded with a teaching stipend for the equivalent of approximately 0.1 full-time equivalent (FTE). This may represent a buy-down of 0.1 FTE, or they may have a full clinical load and the stipend represents a teaching overload. The 0.1 FTE includes both the coaching effort and class time for the PIF course. Coaches receive ongoing faculty development prior to starting work as a coach that continues on regular intervals throughout each semester as part of faculty development meetings. The faculty development process in the inaugural year began with a virtual session led by the faculty from the American Medical Association Coaching program, to set the stage for the conversion from an existing mentoring program to a coaching program. The director of faculty development provides the training sessions for the coaches. These take place both at the start of the year and on an ongoing basis. The faculty development sessions include key topics such as effective facilitation, coaching vs. mentoring, and effective coaching strategies as well as topics that come up during the PIF course or coaching process. Coaches are kept abreast of current events in the students' lives and are provided with updates about the curriculum and school of medicine.

Evaluation

Program Evaluation
The program evaluation is constructed to assess the effect of the coaching program on individual students, the effectiveness and design of the program, achievement of program objectives, and improvement of the quality of the program. Both quantitative and qualitative data are collected and evaluated. Quantitative data assesses factors such as the impact of the coaching program on academic success, lapses of professionalism, and utilization of resources such as wellness programs, counseling services, and academic support services. Focus groups are held with both faculty and students to explore more granular details of program success and areas for improvement.

Student Assessment
Coaches do not evaluate the students, maintaining a neutral and safe space to assist students in reflection and goal setting. Students complete guided reflections at various points during medical school that allow the coach and student to review and discuss professional growth. In order for students to meet expectations, the coaching program requires student participation and completion of required assignments and coursework.

MODEL 2: UNDERGRADUATE MEDICAL EDUCATION PROFESSIONAL DEVELOPMENT COACHING PROGRAM

Micaela Godzich

Description of the Program
At the University of California, Davis, School of Medicine, we developed an academic coaching program for undergraduate medical students after receiving feedback that students did not feel connected to faculty in a meaningful way and wanted more support from faculty in the development of their professional identity.

Program Objectives
1. Improve medical students' feelings of meaningful connection to faculty.
2. Improve faculty support of medical student PIF.
3. Contribute to the development of students' clinical skills.
4. Build an institutional culture of continuous self-improvement through ongoing self-evaluation with the support of trusted faculty.

To address these objectives, we developed a program in which dedicated clinician educator faculty physicians coach individual students longitudinally over the course of their 4 years. Coaches support students both in their individual professional identity development and in the acquisition of the clinical skills needed to become successful physicians without playing a role in their coached students' evaluations.

Coaches interact with students in two distinct ways. They interact with each of their coachees in one-on-one

Vignette 1

Dr. Smith directs the Foundations of Medicine longitudinal preclerkship course, which she developed and implemented during her medical school's curricular renewal. Students have valued the integration of PIF into their preclinical curriculum and clinical skills experiences. However, their evaluations reflect their desire for more individualized guidance about career exploration. They desire an earlier start to "building relationships with faculty." Dr. Smith is eager to develop an individualized coaching program to promote academic, personal, and professional growth. She believes early connectivity with faculty could be the missing link to improve the entire medical student experience. Unfortunately, she hears only about budget cuts due to the expenditures from the curricular renewal. Faculty are already committed facilitators for small group teaching. She worries she would not be able to recruit any faculty coaches or have any resources to devote to faculty development. Unsure about how to frame this idea to her administration, she is struggling to identify the right approach.

Thought Questions

1. What could Dr. Smith do to implement a coaching program with very limited resources? How might she recruit faculty?
2. What specific barriers might she encounter?
3. Who are the key stakeholders to approach with a proposal? What outcomes might provide justification for education leaders to consider this investment?

coaching sessions to guide them in their self-evaluation, identification of challenges and opportunities, and in the design of individual professional development plans with goal setting using the SMART format. In addition, coaches serve as instructors in the clinical skills curriculum, facilitating small groups composed of their own cohort of coaching students. Through this dual role, our coaches contribute to their students' progress in their acquisition of clinical skills and to their professional identity development. This dual role is a deliberate intervention to facilitate a relationship between coach and coachee that is anchored in the shared professional identity of being or becoming a physician. The coaches' demonstration of professional expertise in the group clinical skills sessions with their coaching cohort legitimizes them as clinician educators in the eyes of their coaching students. This proven identity in turn validates the support and feedback coaches provide to students in individual coaching sessions focused on professional identity development.

Program Logistics

Our longitudinal academic coaching program randomly assigns 1 of 16 coaches to each medical student upon matriculation to their first year of medical school. Each coach has an average of 8 students in each year of medical school, with a total of approximately 32 coachees per coach. The 16 coaches are clinical faculty physicians in the school of medicine. The office of medical education funds the coaches' home department 0.2 FTE for the coaching work. The selected coaches come predominantly from primary care disciplines, and approximately 75% are within 5 years of finishing residency.

Coaches are expected to be present at major school events, including induction, match day, and commencement. Social gathering of coaching cohorts is encouraged through financial support of meals; individual coaches host their entire coaching cohorts for a social event twice a year. These meetings of coaching cohorts encourage peer and near-peer support and mentoring within coaching cohorts of students at different stages of training. During the COVID-19 pandemic, this interaction was replaced by virtual participation by coaches in major student events and virtual "happy hours" with student coaching cohorts.

Coaches are required to be available on two predetermined half days per week to consistently facilitate small group clinical skills sessions with each coaching cohort. There are approximately 30 sessions in the first year, 20 sessions in the second year, and 8 sessions in the third year.

These small group sessions are the cornerstone of the longitudinal clinical skills course; coaches guide their coaching student groups through the practice of physical exams and interviewing techniques with standardized patients and review clinical cases to develop clinical decision-making abilities. To avoid coaches having any evaluative role in their coachees' academic career, the students are scored on their acquisition of these skills by other faculty, including other coaches. Coaches administer observed standardized clinical exams (OSCEs) and clinical performance examinations (CPXs) for students who are not in their cohorts.

In addition to these clinical skills sessions, coaches are expected to meet with all of their coachees individually at least three times per year during important transitional times for each cohort of students. Examples of significant times of transition for students include the first month of the first year, before dedicated preparation time for the USMLE Step 1 exam, after their first clinical clerkship in their third year, and early in their fourth year as they plan for residency application.

During individual coaching sessions, coaches and coachees review the student's academic performance through the use of a dashboard that summarizes their academic performance prior to and during medical school. This includes all grades and narrative evaluations from the clerkship years. Coaches support students in continuous self-evaluation and the development of short- and long-term goals using the SMART format. In addition, coaches review their coachees' videos of standardized clinical exams as needed when remediation is indicated to discuss opportunities for improvement.

Coaches also direct their coachees to appropriate resources as indicated and have an ongoing working relationship with providers and staff in the school's wellness office and with the education specialists in the academic support unit. In addition, coaches assist coachees with finding mentors in their specialty of interest.

Coaches document their meetings with coachees in an internal online system that tracks the date of the meetings and includes the ability to describe the meetings in free text and to assign tags to the meetings to designate if they addressed academic issues, personal issues, preparation for standardized tests, professional identity, or other issues. This system is confidential, accessible only to individual coaches and the director of the coaching program, and used to remind coaches of the students' arc throughout their longitudinal relationship. In addition, collection of the tagged data allows for a review of the themes addressed during the individual meetings. This in turn guides faculty development content for coaches.

Faculty Development

Initial faculty development for coaches was provided in the form of an interactive half-day retreat reviewing the structure of the program, the concept of coaching (distinguishing it from mentorship and advising), effective feedback, and working with diverse learners. Thereafter, 90-minute faculty development sessions occur monthly on days when no small group sessions are scheduled. The general structure for these sessions includes discussion of a challenging coaching scenario, followed by invited guests who review school resources and new curricular programming or discussion of concepts in effective coaching. Invited guests have included members of the committee on student progress, the director of the office of wellness, and educational experts from outside institutions. To provide more in-depth faculty development with active participation, we hold twice yearly, half-day retreats. The content includes workshops, coaching program assessment using the SWOT (strengths, weaknesses, opportunities, threats) analysis format, and a shared meal, creating a sense of community among coaches. During the COVID-19 pandemic, all of these meetings continued, taking place on the Zoom video conferencing platform and coaches were provided with DoorDash credit, an online food delivery platform, to order a meal to be eaten during the meetings.

The structure of the program and content of faculty development is designed collaboratively between the associate dean of students and the director of the coaching program. The director of the coaching program is a coach in the program and has an additional 0.2 FTE dedicated to coaching program development and participation in the office of medical education administration. In addition, the program has a dedicated administrative assistant with 0.5 FTE to contribute to the creative development of the program, maintain the coaching website, coordinate meetings, and ensure timely task completion through email reminders to coaches.

Evaluation

The academic coaching program was initially developed in response to graduate questionnaire surveys and is now in its third year of existence. Before implementation of the academic coaching program, graduate questionnaire surveys had reported that a majority of students did not feel a connection with individual faculty members and lacked mentorship (as defined by the Association of American Medical Colleges). Surveys obtained from first- and second-year medical students regarding their satisfaction with coaches were uniformly positive. The current graduate questionnaire responses relevant to contact with faculty were also significantly improved, and we attribute this to the implementation of the program.

Ongoing surveys for students, coaches, and colleagues in the office of medical education document our program's progress and impact. An educational specialist and analyst work with the coaching program leadership to determine the best strategies to track the impact of the coaching program beyond the graduate questionnaire and determine future directions.

MODEL 3: PEER COACHING TO PROMOTE STUDENT SUCCESS

Antwione Haywood

Description of the Program

Conventional student-peer models focus on mentoring and tutoring,[1] whereas models on faculty-student coaching tend to be clearer in the literature than student-driven peer-to-peer models.[2,3] Our student-peer coach at Indiana University School of Medicine is a point person who can offer guidance to peer trainees as they navigate their educational training. Peer coaches act as a neutral party who receive training on coaching their peers through many of the same challenges

Vignette 2

A coachee comes to meet with a peer coach for their fall semester meeting. The coachee reports, "My clinical preceptor told me I need to dress more professionally in the clinic. I don't understand what the big deal is. I think my presentable clothes are fine for the doctor's office. And, with all of my loans, I really can't afford to buy new clothes."

Thought Questions

1. How can the peer coach help the coachee explore the meaning of "professional clothes" and better meet the preceptor's expectations in an equitable way?
2. What are some advantages to having a peer serve as a coach (rather than faculty) in this situation?
3. Are there disadvantages to selecting peers as coaches?

---

they have faced. The goal of a coach is to function as a guide and listener. We encourage the peer coach to believe the coachee is the expert of their own journey and to serve as a thought partner but not as a tutor, adviser, or formal mentor. Our peer coach helps the coachee set and achieve their own academic, social, wellness, and career goals by helping the coachee build self-efficacy and critical thinking skills. Moreover, because students come from all walks of life and may be on a multicampus system, the structured coaching program helps students navigate disparities by improving consistency in experience across campuses.

Program Objectives

1. Improve self-efficacy and success.
2. Provide formal structure for peer-to-peer engagement.
3. Train student leaders in communication and coaching skills.
4. Identify complementary student affairs resources to support the coachee's journey.

Program Logistics

One coach is assigned to six to eight coachees. Coaches are second-year medical students who work with first-year students. They are selected through a two-step interview process and are trained over the summer term. Coaches and coachees participate in an initial get-to-know-each-other meeting during orientation. Subsequently, the pairs have two meetings in the fall semester and one in the spring (more or less based on what works for the coach/coachee pair). Students who don't meet the minimum requirement receive a follow-up email from the student affairs team. Both the coach and coachee sign a coaching agreement that outlines the expectations between the coach and coachee. The coachee completes a set of questions assessing their readiness for coaching. Question 1 asks students to consider areas of growth. Question 2 asks students to reflect on their openness to change. Question 3 asks students to reflect on their own belief that change is possible. These questions are reviewed by the peer coach.

Peer coaches are trained to guide coachees around four pillars: guidance, listening, accountability, and the SUPER Coaching model (described later).

Guidance

The primary job of a peer coach is to guide the coachee toward their own goals. Coaches ask open-ended, thought-provoking questions related to student life (e.g., sense of belonging, connection), academic life (e.g., I'm afraid of failing this class. What should I do?), and personal life (e.g., How do I deal with these feelings of homesickness?). Peer coaching requires one to be a partner by helping coachees learn to find answers to their own questions rather than telling them what to do or jumping to judgment.

Peer coaches are trained to ask the coachee questions about issues they've faced in the past to help prepare them to deal with similar situations in the future and ask questions about problems that have never crossed students' radar. The goal of the questioning process is to elicit the resourcefulness of the coachee. Peer coaches encourage students to seek out answers to their own questions and to connect with the best possible resources, such as faculty advisers or mentors. Generally, a peer coach will work with a student through past reflection on displays of resiliency, resourcefulness, and motivation. Using those themes, the goals of the coach move toward designing future outcomes, discussing barriers, and reframing negative answers toward the positive.

Listener

Listening requires a peer coach to become a generous, nonjudgmental thought partner. A peer coach can offer objective support to coachees by making themselves available with undivided attention. The listening pillar is how coaches develop powerful questions, which often help a coachee get past a barrier, find intrinsic motivation, and solicit resources. For example, if a person is struggling with the idea of not being the top performer, the coach might help the coachee focus on a prior situation in which they had shown a growth mindset in the face of adversity. While listening, the coach is trained to follow these guidelines:

1. Stay out of judgment and enter into every conversation with an open mind. You should try to put yourself in the coachee's shoes, but don't force the coachee into yours.
2. Stay very patient and don't force an outcome that aligns with your thinking. Avoid interruptions, and don't be

afraid to take a moment to collect your thoughts before responding. Silence and wait time are a good listener's best friends.

3. Respond thoughtfully, encouragingly, and directly. When you offer answers, draw direct reference through repetition or restatement to what the speaker was just discussing.

4. Remember what the speaker shared and follow up. If a coachee is really worried about tomorrow's exam, don't forget to ask about it at your next meeting or to shoot them an email to touch base.

Accountability Partner

An accountability partner is not only someone who will always show up prepared, but also someone who will expect others to show up prepared. Peer coaches empower students to remain committed to their own success by helping them set achievable goals and expecting them to meet those objectives. If a student, for example, has a history of not getting enough sleep, peer coaches may review the coachee's sleep schedule with them, ask them to identify clear start and stop times for academic work, help them set up a sleep schedule, and potentially seek additional resources if the sleep issue becomes chronic. Accountability includes planning steps. Coaches are trained to manage accountability with the following guidelines:

The first meeting with the coaching partner should include:

1. Completing a coaching agreement between the coach and coachee partner.
2. Choosing a SMART commitment to accomplish this semester. The SMART goal should be a target behavior the coachee wants to develop, maintain, or decrease.
3. Asking the coachee how the coach can support them in maintaining accountability.

SUPER Coaching

The peer coach works with students with a variety of needs and under many different circumstances. For example, some coachees may wish to focus on academics. Some students may wish to focus on wellness, and some may want to focus on setting and achieving personal goals. In order to examine and address many of these concerns, peer coaches walk students through the SUPER Coaching model. SUPER Coaching allows coaches to help students to create:

1. **S**elf-awareness about what current behavior is taking place
   What's important to you right now?
2. **U**nderstand how that current behavior affects goals
   As opposed to perfect, what would better look like?
3. **P**ropose reinventions of the current behavior by improvement or change
   What do you want to do differently next time?

4. **E**valuate reinvented options
   Which options help you get closer to your goals?
5. **R**eframe gravity (something that weighs heavily on coachee) issues toward the positive rather than the negative and respect boundaries
   How can we move toward something, rather than away from it?

Coachee Responsibility

The coachee is responsible for making a coaching portfolio and is instructed to keep the following items.

- SMART goals
  Specific, measurable, achievable, relevant, time-based
- Progress statements
  Write one or two paragraphs answering the following prompts:
  - Describe whether or not you met your SMART goal and why.
  - Describe whether or not you enjoyed the project.
  - Describe what you learned from your experience working with a coach on the self-management project.

Program Evaluation

The peer-coaching program is measured formally by coachees through evaluation. In general, the focus of the evaluation is on satisfaction, self-reported gains, and usefulness of coaching sessions. In addition, there is general interest in improving academic and social engagement through the peer-coaching program.

Surveys are administered at or near the conclusion of the academic year. The evaluation survey aims to:

- Gather feedback on the effectiveness of and student satisfaction with the peer-coaching program
- Measure how well the program provides students with academic, social, and wellness readiness
- Assess how the program contributes to students' sense of growth and development

MODEL 4: GRADUATE MEDICAL EDUCATION COACHING PROGRAM IN A PEDIATRIC RESIDENCY

Jennifer R. Miller

Description of the Program

In 2013 in response to resident feedback on our traditional faculty adviser system, we developed a longitudinal coaching program that focuses on goal setting and lifelong learning skills for our pediatrics residents. We believe the coaching system helps foster important personal reflection and growth in all aspects of a medical career—beyond just medical knowledge.

Vignette 3

Jeff is a first-year resident and receives an email from his assigned faculty coach asking to schedule his first one-on-one coaching session. He met his coach at intern orientation, and there was never any extra time to reach out to follow up or devote to his self-development. Now, he's on his busiest inpatient month in the intensive care unit (ICU) and feels as though he barely has time to catch up with "life." He has fallen behind with reading or focusing on any in-service exam studying. The last thing he has time for is an additional meeting with a coach. Jeff ignores multiple email reminders and then writes back politely, asking to postpone, citing "no time during my unit month." The coach agrees but asks for a firm date for a meeting. Jeff reluctantly agrees. As the new date approaches, Jeff wishes that these "mandatory meetings" would not be imposed, hoping he could spend any free time sleeping, but he fears reprimand for noncompliance. He begrudgingly agrees to meet.

Thought Questions

1. What might be deterring Jeff from meeting with his coach?
2. Does Jeff's behavior warrant concern? If so, what issues might be concerning?
3. How might the coach be most helpful for Jeff?

Program Objectives

1. Promote individualized learning.
2. Provide a safe space for iterative goal setting and reflection on performance.
3. Facilitate resident wellness and development of skills surrounding burnout prevention.
4. Develop and administer performance improvement plans, when indicated, if academic or professional struggles have reached a threshold at which program leadership has mandated specific action.

Coaches are assigned by residency program leadership, taking into account personalities and core values. Coaches attend a "meet and greet" social function during the resident orientation period, at which time they meet their new residents on a social level. Also during this period, coaches formally meet with their new residents to discuss initial thoughts about strengths, areas for improvement, and long-term goals. Initial topics have included building trust and identifying resident's core values, comparing and contrasting coaching vs. advising, positive psychology philosophy, and assessing professionalism. Because of the COVID-19 pandemic, meetings have been accomplished either in person or via a video platform.

Coaches meet with residents three to four times per year, either in person or virtually, and have access to all resident evaluations and in-training exam scores. This information is used to help the residents identify areas for improvement and develop strategies for success using their areas of strength. Coaches represent a "safe space" for the resident to work on goal setting and individualized curriculum development and discuss feedback, but coaches do not have a summative or evaluative function. In rare circumstances, when a resident requires an official performance improvement plan, the coach is asked to help develop and execute such a plan and then report back to residency leadership about resident progress. These plans vary widely, depending on the area of struggle. Examples would be: clinical skills sessions with live patients, simulation of difficult conversations or specific procedures, discussion of assigned readings on feedback and professionalism, or discussion of specific patient case scenarios.

Program Logistics

Our program has 48 residents and 7 physician coaches from a wide variety of specialties (general pediatrics, pediatric intensive care unit, cardiology, gastroenterology, hospitalist, and endocrinology). One associate program director serves as the lead and contact person responsible for all aspects of the coaching program, including faculty development. Coaches are expected to attend an annual faculty development session (usually 2 hours in the late summer). Coaches are afforded 0.05 FTE (half day every 2 weeks) for their contribution to our program. This FTE was negotiated with our pediatric department chair when the program began.

Program Evaluation

Our coaching program is evaluated formally by residents in an annual program survey. Although feedback has generally been positive, there are always suggestions for improvement. Feedback from the coaches is sought throughout the year during communication with program leadership. So far, we have not formally surveyed our coaches.

Conclusion

We aimed to present various models for coaching in undergraduate and graduate medical education that will encourage future innovations. Establishing an academic coaching program may be a novel way for academic medical center leadership to inspire the next generation of learners and leaders. Through coaching, coaches and coachees can gain valuable skills in listening, reflective practice, and critical thinking. Additionally, programs such as those described can cultivate resilience as an antidote to burnout. These examples elucidate important factors needed to plan, develop, support, implement, and evaluate a successful program.

TAKE-HOME POINTS

1. Developing a coaching program requires adequate resources including faculty time, administrative support, and funding.
2. Faculty development is a critical component of a successful coaching program.
3. Both coaches and coachees must be made fully aware of the goals of the coaching program in order to align expectations and measure outcomes.

QUESTIONS FOR FURTHER THOUGHT

1. What are the best methodologies for evaluation of a coaching program?
2. What is your most significant barrier(s) to developing a coaching program? What might you need to overcome this?

REFERENCES

1. Parsons AS, Kon RH, Plews-Ogan M, Gusic ME. You can have both: Coaching to promote clinical competency and professional identity formation. *Perspect Med Educ.* 2021;10:57–63.
2. Wolff M, Hammoud M, Santen S, et al. Coaching in undergraduate medical education: a national survey. *Med Educ Online.* 2020;25(1).
3. Wolff M, Ross P, Jackson J, et al. Facilitated transitions: coaching to improve the medical school to residency continuum. *Med Educ Online.* 2021;26(1).

10

Developing Coaches for Learners Across the Medical Education Continuum

Sandrijn M. van Schaik, Rebecca Blankenburg, Andrea Marmor, and Caroline E. Rassbach

LEARNING OBJECTIVES

1. Describe the elements of a needs assessment to define the role and responsibilities for coaches in your program and identify resources needed to implement a coaching program.
2. Discuss approaches for recruitment and selection of coaches with attention to diversity and representation.
3. List elements of faculty development for coaches, including onboarding and ongoing skill development to meet the evolving needs of coaches and coachees.
4. Describe common challenges in establishing and maintaining a coaching program and strategies to mitigate these challenges.

CHAPTER OUTLINE

CHAPTER SUMMARY

This chapter provides an overview of the efforts involved in creating a coaching program, with particular emphasis on ensuring coaches are equipped with skills to be effective in their roles. We discuss how a structured approach to program development can help with setting the goal of a coaching program and with choosing a coaching framework to apply to the program. We delineate the elements of a needs assessment to identify the coaching needs of learners in a specific program and identify the resources needed to implement coaching. We describe how to select candidates who will likely be effective in this role and approaches to recruitment that consider diversity and representation. We review the steps toward creating effective faculty development for coaches to help them acquire and maintain essential skills, highlighting the importance of community formation. We also review approaches toward assessment and evaluation of individual coaches and the associated challenges. Lastly, we discuss issues around sustainability of a coaching program and strategies to prevent and mitigate challenges.

INTRODUCTION

Creating a coaching program for learners in medical education is no small undertaking and requires careful planning to ensure the needs of the learners are met and the coaches are set up for success. Coaching is a dynamic activity that requires a variety of skills; thus faculty development is essential for the success of a program. In addition, ongoing support for coaches is needed to help them overcome the challenges that inevitably arise. In this chapter we describe a variety of strategies for creating and supporting a coaching program, illustrated with examples from our own experience and that of others. Many of these strategies

Vignette 1

Jasmine is a program director of an internal medicine residency program at an academic institution. When she reviews annual program evaluation data, she notices that the residents provide low ratings for the feedback they receive. In contemplating this data, she recalls how several faculty members have commented about the decline in longitudinal relationships with residents. As she also noticed a gradual increase in the number of residents who appear to be struggling, she contemplates starting a coaching program. As a first step, she needs to talk to the department chair to obtain buy-in and financial support.

Thought Questions

1. How can the program director make a business case to the department chair?
2. What outcome data should the program collect to demonstrate return on investment?

apply to coaching programs across the continuum, but we will indicate differences between coaching programs for undergraduate medical students versus graduate medical education learners when applicable.

CONCEPTUAL FRAMEWORKS

When designing and implementing a coaching program, we have found it helpful to have a structured approach to ensure the goals are clear to everyone involved and the necessary resources are in place. As coaching may be interpreted differently by different people, choosing a conceptual framework for coaching interactions that aligns with the program's goals is essential. Thus in this section we discuss two types of frameworks: those that can help guide program development and those that guide coaching interactions.

Frameworks to Guide Program Development

A useful framework for initial program development that has been applied to medical education is the logic model. This model is in essence a visual representation of how a program works and the underlying theoretical principles.[1] The model links these principles to program activities and processes, as well as inputs, resources, and program outcomes. The elements of a logic model with an example as applied to a coaching program are summarized in Fig. 10.1. Note that a logic model is not meant to be a detailed implementation plan, rather it is a framework to help with the design of a program, including consideration of assumptions, resources, strategies, and ultimate impact. Detailed guides for using the logic model are available online.[2,3]

Problem statement: With increasing complexity and expansion of medical knowledge, learners need to develop a growth mindset and skills in continuous self-reflection and improvement to achieve required competencies.

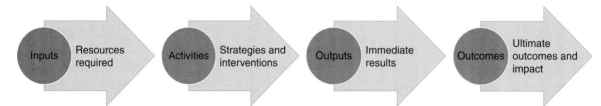

| Inputs | Resources required | Activities | Strategies and interventions | Outputs | Immediate results | Outcomes | Ultimate outcomes and impact |

- Faculty with coaching skills
- Financial support to buy-out time for coaches
- Dedicated time for learners and coaches to meet
- Buy-in from other curricular leaders

- Recruit faculty to the coaching program
- Design and implement faculty development activities for coaches
- Designate time in curriculum for coaching meetings
- Match coaches with learners

- Faculty recruited to program
- Workshops on coaching delivered
- Coaching pairs created
- Coaching meetings conducted

- Learners satisfied with coaching program
- Learners engage in self-reflection
- Learners attain graduation competencies
- Success rate in securing position after graduation increases
- Institution reputation improves
- Match rates increase

Assumptions:
Coaching will be able to foster growth mindset/Learners are interested in developing a relationship with a coach/Our faculty will be able to develop the necessary skills/ . . .

Fig. 10.1 Applying the Logic Model to Planning a Coaching Program.

TABLE 10.1   Application of Kern's Six Steps for Curriculum Development to Planning a Coaching Program

Step	Associated Questions	Rationale
1. Problem identification and general needs assessment	What problem does the coaching program try to solve? For whom? What happens currently, and what is the ideal?	Identifies stakeholders Builds an argument of need Creates an initial understanding of overall goals
2. Targeted needs assessment	What needs do learners have? How would they like to see these needs met? What resources exist?	Informs goals and objectives Ensures learner buy-in Identifies existing resources
3. Goals and objectives	What is the overall program goal? What are the specific (measurable) objectives?	Verifies that the program will solve the problem identified and ensures the learners' needs will be met Informs assessment of outcomes
4. Educational strategies	What conceptual framework for coaching will meet the learners' needs and can accomplish the objectives? What coaching strategies will be employed?	Aligns the conceptual framework and strategies with goals and objectives and learners' needs Informs faculty development for coaches
5. Implementation	How will the program be implemented? Who will do what by when and how?	Guides actual project management Ensures adequate preparation and anticipation of barriers
6. Evaluation	What outcomes will be assessed, when, and by whom?	Verifies that goals and objectives are accomplished Helps build an argument for ongoing program support

Another useful framework is Kern's six steps for curriculum development.[4] Although this model was created to guide the design and implementation of curriculum in medical education, the steps can be applied to the development of a coaching program as well. As illustrated in Table 10.1, the model leads to questions that provide important direction. Note that both the logic model and Kern's six steps start with articulating the problem the program will address, an essential step that should not be skipped. They also both emphasize formulating the desired outcomes (or goals and objectives) up front. The latter provides guidance for identifying which coaching conceptual framework to apply to the program, as we discuss in more detail next.

Lastly, it can be useful to think about change management models when planning a coaching program. For example, although coaching is different from mentoring, this difference may not necessarily be apparent to all stakeholders. If some other form of mentoring or advising program is already in place, the idea that learners may also benefit from coaches may hit resistance. Kotter's eight-step process for leading change provides helpful tips on how to overcome such resistance.[5]

Regardless of the guiding framework used, development and implementation of a coaching program should be seen as an iterative process, with the goal of continuous improvement and adaptation to feedback and changes in the learning environment. Analogous to the Master Adaptive Learner model,[6] described in detail in Chapter 2, ongoing assessment of program outcomes should inform adaptations to program goals, coaching strategies, and coach faculty development (Fig. 10.2).

Frameworks to Guide Coaching Interactions

Choosing a conceptual framework for coaching interactions is an important component of planning the program. Various theoretical frameworks exist that can inform the approach to coaching, as summarized in Chapter 3. The literature also provides examples of models that provide guidance on how to apply theories to coaching interactions, including the Master Adaptive Learner model described in Chapter 2. Other models include the Coaching in Medicine

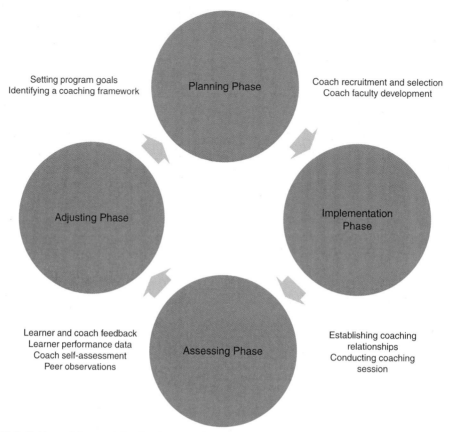

Setting program goals
Identifying a coaching framework

Planning Phase

Coach recruitment and selection
Coach faculty development

Adjusting Phase

Implementation
Phase

Learner and coach feedback
Learner performance data
Coach self-assessment
Peer observations

Assessing Phase

Establishing coaching
relationships
Conducting coaching
session

Fig. 10.2 Taking a Master Adaptive Learner Approach to Continuous Improvement of a Coaching Program.

Vignette 2

Jorge is a new faculty member, 2 years out of residency training, who is applying for a coaching position in a new coaching program for medical students. The position involves clinical and professional skills teaching and advising with a small group of medical students for 4 years. His application shows that he teaches in one of the core science blocks for first year medical students and has received high ratings on evaluations. He also is active on the residency well-being committee and is known to be a strong advocate for learners.

Thought Questions

1. How would you decide if Jorge is qualified?
2. What information about prior experiences would be most relevant? What additional information could you ask for?
3. What would you ask the applicant in order to assess his motivation and preparation for this position?

model[7] and the R2C2 framework,[8] which are described in Chapter 7.

The choice of conceptual framework(s) and model(s) to use should be based on the goals of the coaching program and the needs of the participants. Because coaching programs often seek to address complex educational challenges—such as clinical skills development, communication skills, professional growth, connectedness, or burnout—multiple frameworks should be considered and may often be combined.

In addition to choosing a conceptual framework in which to situate the coaching relationship, we have found it helpful to consider different structural models for coaching as well. Coaching can occur between individuals or within a group and may occur in an isolated meeting or as part of an ongoing, longitudinal relationship. Coaches can be supervisors, peers, or third parties who are neither supervisors nor peers. Coaching programs may employ coaches who work with learners within a defined area in which they have expertise, such as within a specialty or across specialties. The approach depends on the goals of the program and the needs of the learners. For example, many medical student coaching programs have coaches work with small groups of medical students longitudinally over 2 years or longer. These coaches may teach basic clinical skills such as doctor-patient communication, the physical exam, professionalism, and clinical reasoning in addition to providing career advice and mentorship as students explore multiple specialties. At the graduate medical education level, some programs have coaches work longitudinally with residents on core skills such as communication and clinical reasoning, whereas other programs have coaches work with residents on skills specific to clinical practice areas, such as primary care or hospital medicine. Some coaching programs will be designed to foster growth in all learners, whereas others will focus on learners who are struggling or in need of remediation.

CONDUCTING A NEEDS ASSESSMENT

Kern's six-step model distinguishes between two types of needs assessments: a general needs assessment and a targeted needs assessment.[5] A general needs assessment helps distinguish between the current state and the ideal, thereby strengthening the rationale for establishing a coaching program. A general needs assessment may begin with informal discussions with individuals or groups of stakeholders to understand the problems that need solving more clearly. For example, are learners performing suboptimally in a certain area? Are there competencies that could be better taught in the context of a longitudinal relationship, such as communication skills? What other roles might coaches play? This phase of the needs assessment should also include a thorough review of various coaching models and frameworks, such as those already described, to gain understanding of what may work best for a specific coaching program.

A targeted needs assessment involves more in-depth data gathering from key stakeholders through focus groups, interviews, and surveys. Focus groups and interviews allow for open-ended questions and an exchange of ideas, but typically allow only a limited subset of stakeholders' voices to be heard. Surveys, on the other hand, can be used to gather input inclusively from all the stakeholders. Regardless of the data-gathering method, questions can address the nature of the problem, the factors influencing the problem, the key stakeholders' perspectives on how the problem might be addressed, possible roles of the coaches, desired outcomes, and resources needed. The literature contains multiple examples of surveys, focus groups, and interview guides, which can be modified to match a specific program. In addition to informing program development, data from the needs assessment can provide a baseline to measure the success of a coaching program.

RESOURCES NEEDED TO IMPLEMENT A COACHING PROGRAM

As program development begins, securing the necessary resources should be an early consideration. Resources that are likely to be needed include salary support to protect both faculty and administrative time, faculty development materials, and buy-in from any individuals outside of the coaching program whose support is essential for its success. Coaching programs in which coaches spend significant time with learners require salary support to buy out faculty time. The amount of salary support will vary depending on the number of learners per coach and the time required for each learner; amounts between 5% and 25% full-time equivalent are common. A rough estimate applied by the programs at our institutions is 1% to 2% per learner coached. Some programs have volunteer faculty as coaches, which may work well if the expectations about time investment are relatively limited. Peer coaches may not require salary support if the coaching role fits in the workflow of the learner group, for example, peer coaches who are taught to coach one another as part of a clinical experience. Administrative support will be dependent on the scale of the program but should include support for the scheduling of coaching meetings, faculty development, and learner assessment. Faculty development materials may include (paid) courses for coaches, invited speakers, books, and equipment for simulations and role plays. Finally, buy-in from the community is essential to support the program. For example, at the graduate medical education level, faculty buy-in may be required so residents can step away from clinical care for a meeting with their coach.

RECRUITING NEW COACHES

When recruiting new coaches, we believe it is helpful to develop a detailed coaching job description that includes desired skills and prerequisites and a realistic estimate of time commitment and a typical schedule. In general, an application process (rather than appointing coaches) may lead to more dedicated coaches who enter the position fully aware of its requirements. The application process should be standardized and as free of bias as possible. The application might include: a statement of intent/interest (to assess interest and motivation), educational curriculum vitae or educator's portfolio (to assess prior mentoring, feedback, and educational experience), and teaching evaluations and/or recommendations from learners. A structured or semistructured interview process is highly recommended in order to fairly evaluate each potential coach. Interview scenarios or questions could assess interest, motivation, and time to dedicate to the coaching role, along with key

---

Vignette 3

Joy is a medical student coach who is getting burned out because a few of her students phone her regularly. She feels they treat her more like a counselor/best friend/parent than a professional coach. At the same time, she feels other students don't really appreciate her. She feels insecure because other coaches don't seem to have the same issues and wonders whether this is the right role for her.

Thought Questions

1. How would you support this coach? How can a community of practice be promoted to assure support from other coaches?
2. What could be done to clarify the goals of the program, for both learners and coaches, and help a coach set boundaries?

---

coaching skills such as creating a safe environment, providing feedback, and supporting struggling learners. A rating rubric to assign points to different domains for each applicant can be useful in making selection decisions. Just as with workforce and trainee recruitment, recruitment of coaches must include deliberate consideration of diversity and inclusion. Although the benefits of having coaches from diverse backgrounds are not debatable, there is uncertainty about the benefits of matching coaches one-to-one with learners in terms of personal characteristics, career interests, or other factors.

On the one hand, incongruence between mentor and mentee may lead to dissatisfaction. The mentorship literature has shown that the lack of mentor-mentee fit can impede mentee progress, compromise trust, and elicit feelings of vulnerability or isolation in the mentee.[9] In addition, coaches often become role models and, consistent with the professional identity formation conceptual framework described by Cruess et al.,[10] they play an important role in helping learners develop their personal and professional identity. For underrepresented in medicine (UiM) learners in particular, having role models who share their personal characteristics (race/ethnicity, gender, gender identity, sexual orientation, abilities, religion, etc.) has been shown to help with a sense of belonging and influence career choices.[11,12]

On the other hand, it can be argued that exposure to different viewpoints is beneficial to learners. The literature on mentoring in medical education has not revealed substantive evidence that matching mentees to mentors with the same demographic characteristics provides better outcomes, as opposed to matching personality and communication styles.[13] Several programs reported positive outcomes with a random assignment strategy, including increased self-confidence and improved professional and personal development among mentees.[14] Aside from potential benefits and downsides, it simply may not be possible to match coaches and learners based on all characteristics as there continues to be a relative shortage of women in certain fields and of UiM faculty in all of academic medicine.

DEVELOPING EFFECTIVE COACHES

To ensure coaches can be effective in their role, they need to develop and maintain a set of skills or competencies aligned with the coaching model identified for the program. Chapter 4 describes such competencies in detail. Here we discuss the necessary faculty development. As has been described for mentoring, coaching skills are not innate but need to be nurtured and practiced.[15] Kern's six steps, outlined in Fig. 10.2 and described previously as a model to assist with design of the coaching program, can also be used in the design and implementation of coach faculty development.[16] In particular, conducting a targeted needs assessment to understand what skill development prospective coaches in a particular program desire can assist with creating faculty development activities aligned with coaches' skill gaps and preferences. Such a needs assessment can be based on self-assessment, peer review, and/or learner evaluations. It is ideally based on a combination of data sources to avoid blind spots inevitably associated with self-assessment alone. It can be useful to ask coaches about prior formal faculty development in teaching, mentoring, feedback, and other relevant topics to verify understanding of foundational concepts. A targeted needs assessment can also guide the format, timing, and duration of faculty development initiatives, as most coaches will have competing demands on their time and may have different preferences for asynchronous versus in-person learning. Setting goals and objectives, grounded in the desired coach competencies, can further help with deciding on educational strategies, as does the type of content being covered. For example, knowledge and general principles may be more amenable to self-directed reading and other asynchronous strategies than skills, which tend to benefit from experiential strategies. In particular communication skills such as active listening, establishing a relationship, and effective feedback may be best acquired through small group activities such as workshops, case discussions, role-plays, or simulations.[17,18]

When deciding on educational strategies, consider both formal and informal approaches, as learning by doing, observing, and reflecting in the actual workplace can lead to meaningful skill development.[19] Peer observation and "co-coaching" can be helpful, as can the formation of a coach community of practice. A community of practice is defined as "a group of people who share a concern or a passion for something they do and learn how to do it better as they interact regularly."[20] At one institution, formation of a coach community of practice occurred as coaches had informal and formal opportunities to spend time together. These opportunities played an important role in ongoing development and mutual support.[21] In addition, both faculty development and having a community can strengthen coaches' professional identity formation, which helps with recognition, feeling valued, and overall career development.[22]

ASSESSING COACHES AND EVALUATING THE COACHING PROGRAM

To inform ongoing faculty development and to ensure individual coaches indeed have the required competencies, assessing coaches is essential. This can be challenging for various reasons. Although a myriad of data can be collected to inform coach performance evaluations—from learners, the coach, or the coach's peers—each source has limitations. Data obtained from learners can include learner feedback and learner performance over time. Learner feedback is essential, but honest feedback can be difficult to obtain as learners may perceive a power differential and have concerns about sharing feedback that is not positive. Collecting feedback about a coach in aggregate may mitigate this issue, but only if a coach is assigned multiple learners. As coaches typically know their learners well, true confidentiality is challenging even in that scenario. Ensuring that learners understand that coaches want to improve their skills and take a growth mindset approach to feedback can also help with generating honest, constructive feedback.[23]

Another approach is for coaches to ask learners to compare their experience with the coach to other coaching relationships, including those outside of medicine: "What have others done that has worked well for you in a coaching relationship?" Learner performance data can provide further insight into the effectiveness of a coach. Although performance data for an individual learner cannot be directly attributed to a coach, if the same coach has multiple struggling learners who don't seem to be able to overcome their struggles this may be a warning sign about the coach's effectiveness.

Coaches themselves can be another data source: self-assessment and reflection can offer valuable insights on growth edges and challenges. Setting clear expectations and exposing coaches to peers can help provide benchmarks to guide self-assessment, thereby making self-assessment "informed" and more reliable and useful.[24]

A third source of coach performance data can come from peers, through either peer observation or more informal data gathering based on peer interactions with coaches or their learners. Peer observation has been demonstrated to be of great value to teachers in medical education,[25] and for certain coaching interactions scheduled peer observation may be feasible and effective. However, the personal nature of coaching relationships, whether in the one-on-one or small-group setting, may make the more important interactions less amenable to peer observation.

Because of the limitations associated with each of the potential data sources, coach performance evaluation is perhaps best served by a programmatic approach.[26] This approach deemphasizes the importance of the reliability of individual data points in assessment and encourages the collection of multiple different data points that together can create a comprehensive picture of performance. Such data points can be collected on a data dashboard and inform an individual development plan for coaches, mimicking performance assessment and learning plans used with clinicians and learners.[27,28] Whether such a programmatic approach to assessment is feasible and acceptable in the context of coaching deserves further study. In addition, further exploration of ways to determine whether coaching programs have the desired outcomes is needed. This, and other gaps in the literature around coaching in medical education, is discussed in more detail in Chapter 3. Regardless of the approach to coach performance evaluation, the primary goal should be to create a plan for improvement and further growth. Coaches require coaching themselves, and careful consideration of how coaches can be supported in their own ongoing growth and development is essential for the success of a program.

In the next section, we discuss typical challenges in coaching and ways in which coaches can be supported to overcome such challenges. Setting expectations up front and creating transparent processes for coaches who are not meeting expectations is essential.

CHALLENGES FOR COACHES AND COACHING PROGRAMS AS WELL AS MITIGATION STRATEGIES

Even with the best possible preparation and attention to the frameworks covered in the previous sections, coaching programs and coaches are bound to run into difficulties. Although some of these difficulties can be avoided with careful planning, expecting challenges to occur and developing a system to recognize them and intervene early provides the best chance of course correction. It may not feel that way at the time, or for all involved, but each challenge represents an opportunity for growth and development and ultimately improvement and customization of the program. Our experience suggests that challenges tend to fall into several broad categories. Table 10.2 describes

TABLE 10.2   Common Challenges in Coaching Programs With Mitigation Strategies

Challenge ⇩ Possible Impact if Not Addressed	Subcategories With Examples	Mitigation Strategies
Inadequate coach preparation ⇩ <ul><li>Coaches unable to meet learners' needs</li><li>Coach burnout/dropout</li><li>Learners experience disparities in coaching experience</li></ul>	Content of training inadequate to meet coaching needs *e.g., A learner confides in their coach about unusual circumstances (disability, family stressors, medical illness) that the coach feels unprepared to handle* Coach training needs are asynchronous with scheduled faculty development *e.g., A learner has academic needs/ questions that come up before those topics have been covered in coach faculty development* Content of training does not feel targeted to coach's diverse skill sets, strengths, and needs *e.g., Coaches attend coach orientation and twice-yearly faculty development but feel that sessions are either too advanced or too basic for their needs* Difficulty coordinating faculty development with faculty schedules *e.g., Program experiences dwindling attendance at coach faculty development sessions*	<ul><li>Provide both synchronous and asynchronous learning</li><li>Robust, organized, and accessible platform for storing training materials</li><li>Consider smaller group trainings for specific skill sets (e.g., cohort coaches by specialty for clinical skills training)</li><li>Recognize boundaries of what is and isn't the responsibility of the coach to know and when to refer out</li><li>Have coach experts participate in design of training activities</li><li>Make leadership accessible for as-needed training/support needs</li><li>Make sure that in-person, on-time sessions are high yield</li><li>Ensure that clear expectations of roles and boundaries of coach responsibilities are included in coach training</li><li>Periodic high-yield skills refreshers throughout the year</li><li>Coordinate training with upcoming needs—provide training "just in time"</li><li>Ensure coaches have protected time/salary support for faculty development</li></ul>
Problems with coach recruitment ⇩ <ul><li>Coaches are not adequately qualified to meet learners' needs</li><li>Coaches do not match the diversity of identities, backgrounds, and interests of learners</li><li>Poor retention of faculty in coaching program</li></ul>	Inadequate faculty interest or qualified applicants *e.g., Program puts out a call for applicants for a new coaching program, but very few apply*	<ul><li>Feature coaching as a unique part of the curriculum in external and internal newsletters/marketing materials to convey that coaching is valued at the highest levels</li><li>Engage departmental leadership in coach recruitment</li><li>Explicitly invite faculty from specific backgrounds to apply</li><li>Create a rubric to rate applicants against predefined criteria</li><li>Provide additional mentorship for new coaches from less represented backgrounds</li></ul>

TABLE 10.2 Common Challenges in Coaching Programs with Mitigation Strategies—cont'd		
Challenge ⇩ **Possible Impact if Not Addressed**	**Subcategories With Examples**	**Mitigation Strategies**
	Lack of diversity of background, gender, ethnicity, specialty, etc., in applicants *e.g., The first round of applicants for a student coaching program are qualified, but most are white women in general medical fields*	
	Disagreement or inconsistency about what skills/qualities are necessary in a coach *e.g., The recruitment committee struggles to agree on which applicants to accept, with some prioritizing teaching experience, whereas others prioritize clinical skills*	
Balancing coaching with other priorities ⇩ • Program unable to recruit coaches from certain specialties • Perceived inequity in expectations between coaches from different specialties • Poor retention of faculty in coaching program	Coaching demands conflict with clinical or academic expectations *e.g., Several coaches quit because their coaching duties conflict with their division's expectations for clinical work and attendance at national meetings* Coaches from certain specialties less able to attend coaching or faculty development activities *e.g., Coaches from procedural specialties feel pressure from their department to stop coaching because of the difficulty in scheduling operating room time around their coaching schedule* Disparities in coach absences *e.g., An administrator notices that some coaches request twice as many absences than other coaches, citing clinical duties*	• Clear expectations up front at recruitment about time commitment and expectations for attendance • When possible, identify options for flexibility of timing/location of coaching sessions • Solicit coach nominations/letters of support from less represented departments/divisions to encourage buy-in • Leadership could offer to advocate for coach with their departments/divisions • Consider having coaches in high-demand specialties cover for each other • Plan for additional coverage/flexibility for times of year with high coach absences • Involve coaches in identifying solutions to conflicting priorities

Continued

TABLE 10.2	**Common Challenges in Coaching Programs With Mitigation Strategies—cont'd**	
Challenge ⇩ **Possible Impact if Not Addressed**	**Subcategories With Examples**	**Mitigation Strategies**
Loss of support from health system, institution, or learners ⇩ Lack of sustainability of program • Inability to show positive impact of program • Inability to secure funding for future coaching endeavors	Resistance from other teaching and nonteaching faculty *e.g., A group of noncoach faculty complains to their department that they are also spending significant time teaching and mentoring learners but are not afforded protected time* Loss of funding for coaching program *e.g., In response to budget cuts, funding for a successful coaching program is unexpectedly cut off* Lack of support from learners *e.g.. A group of learners complain to leadership that scheduled coaching activities are taking time away from other clinical/learning opportunities*	• Build a plan to collect information on impact of program into the program design • Collect and document evidence of learner buy-in—a very powerful motivator for learning institutions • Document patient buy-in/impacts if possible • Periodically provide metrics of coach performance (evidence of training, time spent coaching, assessments of their coaching) to each coach and division/department head, to support their recognition and promotion
Interpersonal mismatch/conflict ⇩ • Breakdown of trust between coach and learners • Perceived inequity between coach's individual learners • Coach unable to meet learners' needs • Coach burnout	Coaching group dynamics *e.g., A coaching group is divided on whether a group project has educational value, and work is unequally distributed as a result* Coaches' expertise does not match that of learner *e.g., A learner has very specific career aspirations and clinical skill needs that do not match the coach's areas of expertise* Breakdown of trust between learner and coach *e.g., A learner goes to coaching leadership stating that they feel their coach is not supportive of their needs and they would like a new coach* Coach struggles to support a particular learner *e.g., Coach approaches leadership feeling conflicted about whether a learner's advocacy efforts are detrimental to the group's ability to focus on clinical skills during teaching sessions*	• Set clear expectations (and limits) for coach role and learner role—revisit and reemphasize throughout the coaching cycle • Anticipate and normalize healthy conflict, along with a clear plan for addressing it • Provide a clear set of procedures for addressing concerns • Leadership could proactively check in with coaches and learners throughout the coaching cycle to identify concerns and address them early • Train coaches in skills of resilience and self-care in the face of interpersonal conflict • Provide training in evidence-based communication strategies around managing and resolving conflict

TABLE 10.2	**Common Challenges in Coaching Programs With Mitigation Strategies—cont'd**	
Challenge ⇩ **Possible Impact if Not Addressed**	**Subcategories With Examples**	**Mitigation Strategies**
Threats to coach well-being ⇩ • Coaches' mental and physical health suffers • Poor retention of coaches in program • Reputation of coaching program suffers • Difficult to recruit new coaches	Coaches feel overwhelmed by coaching role *e.g., A coach feels a learner who is leaning on them for emotional support is affecting their own relationship* Coaches don't feel adequately supported by the coaching program *e.g., A group of coaches approaches leadership stating the program does not adequately consider the needs of coaches with children* Coaches feel isolated *e.g., Coaches in a large academic center rarely encounter other coaches, as they are in different departments and campuses*	• Create regular peer check-ins just for coaches—ideally incorporated into coaching schedule • Provide training and reinforcement of skills in setting and maintaining boundaries and balance • Create a peer support/buddy program • Online forum for coaches to share difficulties and how they approached them • Clear messaging of role of program leadership in the event of conflict between coaches and learners • Provide a confidential "coach advocate" to whom coaches can go to with concerns • Prioritize coach community building by scheduling it into coaching calendar

some common types of challenges that coaching programs and coaches may experience and suggests some initial approaches to address them. Table 10.3 contains additional tips and best practices to prevent challenges.

Any of these challenges, if not addressed, may threaten sustainability of the coaching program. Several of the key steps covered earlier in this chapter can help protect program sustainability when challenges arise. At the beginning

TABLE 10.3	**Additional Tips to Prevent Common Challenges**	
Tips for Success	**Practical Application/Examples**	**Possible Benefits**
Communicate clear expectations to coaches and those who support them.	• Clear and detailed job description • Routine and explicit communication between coaching leadership and coaches' departments about expectations for coaching, early in recruitment • Ask coach's department to sign a letter or statement of support for coach	• Allows applicants to realistically assess their ability to join the coaching program • Decreases sense of inequity between coaches • Improves retention • Improves buy-in of key stakeholders
Encourage coaches to set norms, boundaries, and expectations early and often.	• Build in time early in coaching relationship specifically for this process • Build in time to revisit these norms throughout the coaching relationship • Set some programmatic expectations, and allow coaching groups some flexibility within limits	• Encourages learners and coaches to take ownership for their relationship • Gives coaches and learners a standard to refer to when conflict occurs • Normalizes the evolution and reassessment of the coaching relationship over time

Continued

TABLE 10.3   Additional Tips to Prevent Common Challenges—cont'd

Tips for Success	Practical Application/Examples	Possible Benefits
Make coach well-being a priority from the beginning.	• Schedule coach activities into calendar that focus primarily on community building and getting to know each other • Minimize required coach activities outside of scheduled coaching day/time • Consider a formal coach support system, such as a buddy program • Provide adequate coverage for family leave, vacation, etc.	• Reduces isolation, burnout • Models lifelong skills for learners • Improves retention • Assures recruitment of a diverse and talented coaching pool
Check in proactively with coaches and learners at expected intervals.	• Routine biannual check-in from leadership about coaching relationship • Provide a confidential, accessible, and supportive outlet for learners to discuss concerns • Regular coach self-assessment and learner evaluations, reviewed by leadership for identification of early concerns	• Detects issues early with opportunity to intervene • May prevent deterioration of relationships, including possible coach drop-out or dismissal
Encourage a growth mindset in both coaches and learners by normalizing challenges and a process for addressing them.	• Schedule time regularly into coaching sessions for coach to ask for feedback or suggestions (could use a framework such as "keep-start-stop") • Coaches meet with peers regularly to informally discuss challenges and support each other • Provide a clear and supportive method for identifying and responding to concerns from coaches and learners	• Establishes essential habits of reflection, cultural humility, and lifelong learning • Strengthens bonds between coaches and learners • Reflects and models lifelong continuous improvement
Build in flexibility around timing and location of coaching interactions as along with faculty development whenever possible	• Provide faculty development in multiple formats: scheduled, asynchronous, and "just in time" • Ask qualified coaches who decide not to apply because of time constraints, "What would make you able to play this role?" • When coaching sessions are in-person, rationale and benefits should be clear to coach and to learners. • Offer options to conduct coaching sessions in remote and asynchronous formats when appropriate	• Increases diversity of coaching pool • Increases satisfaction of coaches and learners • Enhances participation of learners and coaches with time, location, or ability constraints

of this chapter, we discussed the importance of a strong problem statement to obtain stakeholder buy-in. Equally imperative is the collection of data to demonstrate return on investment, as institutional leadership may otherwise see a coaching program as a nice "extra" that might be the first to get cut when finances are tight. Such data can include learner outcomes and testimonials by learners and coaches as well as other evidence that the coaching program has an impact on the learning environment. Coaches can be role models for other faculty and be champions for change in clinical learning environments.

In addition, anticipating or preventing prolonged coach absences and turnover are essential to ensuring sustainability. As coaching depends on formation of a relationship between the coach and the learner, anything that interrupts the relationship can be detrimental. Yet coaches, like all faculty, may need parental or medical leave or may move on to different roles or different institutions. Depending on the program, sustainability can be protected by building in a coverage plan such as allowing coaches to "cross-cover" for each other during leaves or identifying faculty with experience in other mentoring roles who can be oriented to the coach job to serve as a back-up.

CONCLUSION

Creating and sustaining a coaching program is no small undertaking. Thoughtful planning using a structured approach to set clear goals, identify necessary resources, and create a plan to help coaches develop the skills needed to be effective are all essential to ensure a program's success. Anticipating inevitable challenges and designing a systematic approach to address such challenges is vital. In addition to following the steps proposed in this chapter, it can be incredibly useful to consult with faculty at other institutions that have been successful in setting up a coaching program.

TAKE-HOME POINTS

1. Performing a thoughtful needs assessment will lead to a more successful, targeted coaching program.
2. Coaches' faculty development and community building are essential to sustainability, including ongoing skill development to meet the needs of coaches and the learners and developing a community of medical educators to work through challenges and provide peer support.
3. Though there are common challenges in coaching, strategies exist to mitigate these challenges.

QUESTIONS FOR FURTHER THOUGHT

1. What knowledge, skills, and/or attitudes would your learners benefit most from being coached on, and what coaching model(s) would work best for your learners?
2. What data are you collecting to demonstrate that your coaches and your coaching programs are successful?
3. What challenges do you anticipate encountering, and what strategies will you employ to mitigate those challenges?

ANNOTATED BIBLIOGRAPHY

Rassbach CE, Blankenburg R. A novel pediatric residency coaching program: outcomes after one year. *Acad Med.* 2018;93(3):430–434.
In this paper, the authors provide an exemplar of a coaching program for graduate medical education learners. They describe how they developed and implemented the program and the outcomes they measured to document its success.

Thomas PA, Kern DE, Hughes MT, Chen BY. *Curriculum development for medical education: a six-step approach.* Baltimore: John Hopkins University Press; 2016.
The six-step model for curriculum development can also be applied to the development of a coaching program, as described in this chapter. The book provides in-depth examples to guide the reader through each of the six steps.

van Schaik SM. Accessible and adaptable faculty development to support curriculum reform in medical education. *Acad Med.* 2021;96(4):495–500.
Coaching is a relatively new concept for medical educators and requires faculty development to ensure that new coaches have the necessary skills. This paper provides suggestions for approaches to faculty development in the context of a new program or curriculum.

REFERENCES

1. Savaya R, Waysman M. The logic model: A tool for incorporating theory in development and evaluation of programs. *Adm Soc Work*. 2005;29(2):85–103.
2. Logic Models. Center for Disease Control and Prevention. Program Performance and Evaluation Office. https://www.cdc.gov/eval/tools/logic_models/index.html Accessed August 1, 2021.
3. Logic models for program design, implementation, and evaluation: Workshop toolkit: United States Department of Education Institute of Education Sciences; May 2015. https://files.eric.ed.gov/fulltext/ED556231.pdf Accessed August 1, 2021.
4. Thomas PA, Kern DE, Hughes MT, Chen BY. *Curriculum development for medical education: a six-step approach*. Baltimore: John Hopkins University Press; 2016.
5. Kotter JP, Rathgeber H. *Our iceberg is melting: Changing and succeeding under any conditions*. New York: Macmillan; 2006.
6. Cutrer WB, Miller B, Pusic MV, et al. Fostering the development of master adaptive learners: a conceptual model to guide skill acquisition in medical education. *Acad Med*. 2017;92(1):70–75.
7. Rassbach CE, Blankenburg R. A novel pediatric residency coaching program: outcomes after one year. *Acad Med*. 2018;93(3):430–434.
8. Sargeant J, Lockyer J, Mann K, et al. Facilitated reflective performance feedback: developing an evidence-and theory-based model that builds relationship, explores reactions and content, and coaches for performance change (R2C2). *Acad Med*. 2015;90(12):1698–1706.
9. Koopman RJ, Thiedke CC. Views of family medicine department chairs about mentoring junior faculty. *Med Teach*. 2005;27(8):734–737.
10. Cruess RL, Cruess SR, Boudreau JD, Snell L, Steinert Y. A schematic representation of the professional identity formation and socialization of medical students and residents: a guide for medical educators. *Acad Med*. 2015;90(6):718–725.
11. Dixon G, Kind T, Wright J, Stewart N, Sims A, Barber A. Factors that influence underrepresented in medicine (UIM) medical students to pursue a career in academic pediatrics. *J Natl Med Assoc*. 2020;113(1):95–101.
12. Yehia BR, Cronholm PF, Wilson N, et al. Mentorship and pursuit of academic medicine careers: a mixed methods study of residents from diverse backgrounds. *BMC Med Educ*. 2014;14(1):26.
13. Hee J, Toh YL, Yap HW, et al. The development and design of a framework to match mentees and mentors through a systematic review and thematic analysis of mentoring programs between 2000 and 2015. *Mentor Tutoring: Partnersh Learn*. 2020;28(3):340–364.
14. Tan YS, Teo SWA, Pei Y, et al. A framework for mentoring of medical students: thematic analysis of mentoring programmes between 2000 and 2015. *Adv Health Sci Educ Theory Pract*. 2018;23(4):671–697.
15. Ramani S, Gruppen L, Kachur EK. Twelve tips for developing effective mentors. *Med Teach*. 2006;28(5):404–408.
16. van Schaik SM. Accessible and adaptable faculty development to support curriculum reform in medical education. *Acad Med*. 2021;96(4):495–500.
17. Steinert Y, Mann K, Centeno A, et al. A systematic review of faculty development initiatives designed to improve teaching effectiveness in medical education: BEME Guide No. 8. *Med Teach*. 2006;28(6):497–526.
18. Kopechek J, Bardales C, Lash AT, Walker Jr C, Pfeil S, Ledford CH. Coaching the coach: A program for development of faculty portfolio coaches. *Teach Learn Med*. 2017;29(3):326–336.
19. Steinert Y. Faculty development: from workshops to communities of practice. *Med Teach*. 2010;32(5):425–428.
20. Wenger E. *Communities of practice: Learning, meaning, and identity*. Cambridge, UK: Cambridge University Press; 1999.
21. Sheu L, Hauer KE, Schreiner K, van Schaik SM, Chang A, O'Brien BC. A friendly place to grow as an educator": a qualitative study of community and relationships among medical student coaches. *Acad Med*. 2020;95(2):293–300.
22. Steinert Y, O'Sullivan PS, Irby DM. Strengthening teachers' professional identities through faculty development. *Acad Med*. 2019;94(7):963–968.
23. Anderson L, Silet K, Fleming M. Evaluating and giving feedback to mentors: new evidence-based approaches. *Clin Transl Sci*. 2012;5(1):71–77.
24. Sargeant J, Armson H, Chesluk B, et al. The processes and dimensions of informed self-assessment: a conceptual model. *Acad Med*. 2010;85(7):1212–1220.
25. Hyland KM, Dhaliwal G, Goldberg AN, Chen L-m, Land K, Wamsley M. Peer review of teaching: insights from a 10-year experience. *Med Sci Educ*. 2018;28(4):675–681.
26. Schuwirth LW, Van der Vleuten CP. Programmatic assessment: from assessment of learning to assessment for learning. *Med Teach*. 2011;33(6):478–485.
27. Boscardin C, Fergus KB, Hellevig B, Hauer KE. Twelve tips to promote successful development of a learner performance dashboard within a medical education program. *Med Teach*. 2018;40(8):855–861.
28. Dowding D, Randell R, Gardner P, et al. Dashboards for improving patient care: review of the literature. *Int J Med Inform*. 2015;84(2):87–100.

Coaching Assessment and Program Outcomes

Richard N. Van Eck, Elza Mylona, and Basim Dubaybo

LEARNING OBJECTIVES

1. Define the types, purposes, and activities of program evaluation.
2. Define the four levels of Kirkpatrick's evaluation model.
3. Demonstrate real-world applications of Kirkpatrick's model to the evaluation of coaching programs.
4. Demonstrate evaluation activities outlined in this chapter.
5. Generate an evaluation plan for a coaching program using Kirkpatrick's evaluation model.
6. Generate a plan for calculating return on investment for coaching programs.

CHAPTER OUTLINE

CHAPTER SUMMARY

Because coaching is a process that naturally adapts to different goals, outcomes, and contexts (depending on the coaches and those they are coaching), coaching programs have the potential to improve every aspect of an organization. However, if not designed or implemented effectively, they become a financial, time, and productivity drain.[1] Program evaluation is a critical tool for ensuring your coaching program is having the maximum effect on the organization.[1-2] In this chapter, we show how anyone can apply the basic principles of evaluation to coaching programs to measure their impact, justify the investment, seek continued or additional funding, and make adjustments when necessary.

INTRODUCTION

Coaching programs, when designed and implemented well, require significant resources and financial and time commitments for organizations. It is only reasonable to expect that we will be asked at some point to show the effect of the programs on individuals and the organization overall. The leadership and financial realities that allow for the design and implementation of such programs can change almost overnight, as we have seen as the result of the COVID-19 pandemic in 2020, leading to sudden demands to justify the resources needed. The good news is that program evaluation is a powerful tool for answering this question, and it can be easily employed. However, doing so requires understanding that evaluation is not the last thing we do after the implementation of our coaching programs—it is a necessary corequisite of good program design from the beginning.

Although program evaluation is its own field of study, with dozens of models and approaches, all program evaluation models share core principles and activities that can be mastered and employed to good effect by those who design coaching programs. We highlight these core principles and activities and provide an overview of one of the most powerful and easy-to-use program evaluation tools: Kirkpatrick's four levels of evaluation. Although this chapter is not intended to make the reader an evaluation expert, it will provide a framework to help effectively evaluate, refine, and justify a coaching program.

There are many types of program evaluations, including needs assessment, cost-benefit analysis, formative or summative evaluation, efficiency, process, and outcomes to name just a few. In this chapter, we describe the six most common activities shared by all evaluations to help guide the evaluation of a coaching program. We then provide an overview of three common types of evaluation: outcomes-based evaluation, goal-based evaluation, and process-based evaluation. Each type is designed to examine different components of a coaching program, so it is important to understand which is most appropriate for an individual program's purposes. We then provide an overview of Kirkpatrick's evaluation model and demonstrate how to apply its principles to any evaluation plan. Finally, we outline some of the pitfalls and critical considerations of evaluating coaching programs and include real-world examples.

THREE COMMON TYPES AND PURPOSES OF PROGRAM EVALUATION

Program evaluation is defined as the systematic collection and analysis of information related to the design, implementation, and outcomes of a program for the purpose of monitoring and improving its quality and effectiveness.[3] Most educators assume that one first designs the program and then, later, evaluates it. This is a fundamental and persistent misconception about how evaluation is best done. Ideally, design and evaluation should occur simultaneously, so they are aligned from the start. This can help reveal and address any imperfections in program design or implementation. Information should be collected systematically and deliberately, following the same rigorous methods applied in other types of research, to identify whether the program is effective and what contributes to the success of the program.[4] In simpler terms, we conduct program evaluations to demonstrate program effectiveness (e.g., to funders), to improve the implementation and effectiveness of a program (e.g., to manage limited resources), to justify continued funding, to satisfy ethical responsibility to clients, or to document program development and activities to help ensure successful replication.

Goal-Based Evaluations

These types of evaluations look at the extent to which the coaching program has met its predetermined goals or objectives. They do not evaluate whether the goals themselves are valid, or whether the appropriate measures of effectiveness are being used. Goal-based evaluation

---

Vignette 1

Vickie Reardon was hired 6 months ago as the dean for faculty development at a state-funded medical school. In addition to the usual in-person and online resources for faculty, her portfolio includes a coaching program designed by a former faculty member in which faculty who are great teachers serve as coaches for the junior faculty to develop into effective educator-scholars.

The dean meets with Vickie and informs her that the school has taken a financial hit during the COVID-19 pandemic. "You know that I feel the coaching program is critical to the school and that its expenses are justified," the dean says when they meet, "but I have to look at every department and program and provide evidence for their continued funding. If you can just pull some data together to show its impact, I'm sure we can justify its continuation." Vickie concurs with the dean's assessment—as a certified coach with numerous publications on coaching programs, she knows the program is well-designed and implemented.

Thought Questions
1. What kind of data can Vickie produce to show the program's effectiveness?
2. Asking for evidence of program effectiveness in a crisis suggests the evidence is not routinely evaluated or even collected. If the program is preserved moving forward, how would one establish which data should be routinely collected?
3. How could one prevent being in this precarious position with current or new coaching programs that are developed?

questions include questions such as: How were the goals of the program established? Was the process effective? If not, why? What is the status of the program's progress toward achieving its goals? Do the people involved in the program have adequate resources (time, training, facilities, and budget) to achieve the goals?

Process-Based Evaluations

Process-based evaluations focus on the program's activities rather than its outcomes and offer insight into the program's implementation and management. Activities may include the types and quantities of services delivered, the beneficiaries of those services, the resources used to deliver the services, the practical problems encountered, and the ways such problems were resolved. Process evaluation questions may include: Was the coaching program successful? If so, how and why? What were the kinds of problems encountered in delivering the program? Was the program well managed? Were participants trained or educated to the right level for the program? Was there adequate support (administrative, technical, financial) for the program?

Outcomes-Based Evaluations

Outcome evaluation is the most commonly requested evaluation by accrediting bodies because it establishes whether the program is producing the desired change. It focuses on what changed for program participants and how much difference those changes in turn made for them and the organization. An outcomes-based evaluation is also critical if the organization intends to calculate the return on investment. Outcomes-based questions may include: Did the coaching program succeed in helping students transition to residency? Was the program more successful with certain groups of students or specialties than with others? What aspects of the program did participants say gave them the greatest benefit?

Despite the differences among the three types of evaluations listed, most program evaluations will need to answer questions from all three types. What is most important to remember is that each kind of question is different and requires attention as a part of a full program evaluation. In addition to sharing questions from all three types, program evaluations are also likely to employ the same six activities.

THE SIX ACTIVITIES SHARED BY ALL EVALUATIONS

It is not necessary to master all the intricacies of each evaluation type, but it is important to determine which one is most relevant to the purpose of each program, keeping in mind that it is common to have more than one purpose.

Vignette 2

In response to her dean's request for the effectiveness of the school's coaching program, Vickie compiles a report showing the number of faculty who have been trained as coaches, the number of people who have been coached, the hours of training developed and implemented, the posttraining satisfaction surveys, and the annual reports showing the self-reported data on the effect of the program on teaching practice. The Likert-type data and descriptive statistics paint a portrait of an evidence-based, popular program that has reached a majority of the faculty—the program appears to be on very solid ground.

Thought Questions

1. Is the data presented here evidence of primarily goal-based, process-based, or outcome-based evaluation?
2. What additional data could be provided to represent the three evaluation types?

Regardless of the purpose, all program evaluations share six common activities (see Table 11.1).[5] These activities can serve as a guide in structuring the evaluation process.

Activity One: Posing Questions About the Program

Program evaluation starts with one or more questions, sometimes simple and easy to answer but more often complex (see Table 11.2 for common examples). A good place to start is by asking questions such as: Why do we want to evaluate this program? How will we use the results? What are the evaluation goals of the stakeholders? What will tell us whether the program is performing as designed?

Answers to these questions provide qualitative and quantitative data about how the program adds value to various stakeholders. The answers identify the value of

TABLE 11.1 Typical Program Evaluation Activities
Common Evaluation Activities
1. Posing questions about the program
2. Setting standards for effectiveness
3. Designing the evaluation and selecting the participants
4. Collecting data
5. Creating/assembling relevant expertise
6. Analyzing data and reporting results

TABLE 11.2   Common Program Evaluation Questions
1. To what extent did the program achieve its goals and objectives?
2. For which individuals or groups was the program more effective?
3. What are the characteristics of the individuals or groups who participated?
4. How enduring were the effects?
5. Which features (activities, settings, management strategies) of the program were most/least effective?
6. To what extent are the program's objectives and activities applicable to other settings/institutions?
7. What are the relationships between the cost and the effects of the program?
8. To what extent did changes in social, financial, political, etc., circumstances influence the program's support and outcomes?

the program to the academic mission of the organization. They also outline the effects on the careers of the coachees. Finally, the answers may show how efficiently the program was conducted to yield cost-effective outcomes. As we consider the program's benefits or outcomes, we recommend separating the tangible, such as better performance, increased satisfaction, improved motivation, or decreased conflict, from the intangible, such as increased self-esteem, teamwork, collaboration, contentment with role, or satisfaction with career direction, and try to evaluate both. Intangible outcomes are always more difficult to assess but remain crucial when considering the impact of the coaching program on the bottom line.

Activity Two: Setting Standards for Effectiveness

Program evaluations are concerned with evidence of program effectiveness. Programs are often measured against particular standards; the more specific the standards are, the easier they are to measure. Evaluators must clearly define all potentially ambiguous terms (e.g., high-risk students) in the evaluation questions and standards. For example, if the evaluation question is: Did the first-year students who participated in the coaching program maintain what they learned by the end of their second year? The standard might be: No decreases in learning will be found between students' second and first years. A useful way to think about standards is to decide whether we want to

measure the program's effectiveness in terms of the structure, process, or outcomes of the program. Standards can be established by reviewing other comparable programs, reviewing the literature, or relying on the consensus of experts. Where no clear standards exist, they can be established internally by a careful consideration of the goals and objectives of the program. The challenge is to identify or create standards that are credible, appropriate, and measurable.

Real-World Example

The office of faculty development at a medical school launches a 16-month coaching program. The program is designed to equip midcareer faculty with a deeper awareness of health care operations and to develop relevant leadership skills. In addition to pairing participants with a senior faculty coach, the program offers a professional development seminar series and several networking events. In this scenario, one of the evaluation questions might seek to answer whether participants of the program were successful in assuming leadership positions within their own health care system. The standard of effectiveness for such a question might be that 90% of participants in the new coaching program will seek leadership positions within the organization after a year of completing the program, and 75% will move into the leadership positions for which they apply.

Activity Three: Designing the Evaluation and Selecting the Participants

Ideally, program evaluation should be considered concurrently with design of the coaching intervention, as one can influence the other. Standard evaluation designs include comparing one group's performance over time (when all participants have received the same training) or comparing two groups at one or more times (when some participants receive a different program or no program at all). Some of the general questions to consider at this point may include the following: How many measurements should I make? When should the measurements be made? How should the groups or individuals be chosen?

Activity Four: Collecting Data

The process of collecting and measuring information on variables of interest enables leaders to answer stated research questions, test hypotheses, and evaluate outcomes. Some general principles to consider include finding out what data are already being collected, keeping the evaluation questions front and center to ensure only the necessary data are collected, collecting data from more than one source for each question, and collecting a mix of quantitative and qualitative data. Quantitative data are useful for discovering the magnitude of a phenomenon (e.g., outcomes, barriers, facilitators). Qualitative data are useful to better understand the phenomenon (e.g., who benefits most from a program, what additional support is needed to improve outcomes). Some of the most common sources are direct observations, self-assessments, surveys, interviews/focus groups, existing data (e.g., performance tests), and peer evaluations. Creating an evaluation matrix is a useful tool for keeping track of the methods being considered for collecting data. In its simplest form, a matrix displays evaluation questions in alignment with the data collection strategies that will be used to answer them.

We also recommend that coaching program evaluation includes the perspective of the coach, as it can add valuable knowledge about the coaching relationship and individual outcomes. Because coaching experiences are individual and personal, the evaluation should also include attitude questionnaires with rating scales that capture both positive and negative perceptions and face-to-face interviews and focus group discussions that allow for more comprehensive exploration.[6] Although all of these activities so far are important and collecting data sounds simple, this may be the most important activity of them all.

There are also some common challenges associated with initial data collection. Table 11.3 presents some of the most common challenges we've seen and some of the strategies we've used for addressing them.

Activity Five: Creating/Assembling Relevant Expertise

Program evaluation is a multifaceted process, and the scale and complexity of a coaching program affects the expertise and resources needed. One often overlooked resource is an instructional designer (ID). An ID is an expert who understands how to classify outcomes, generate measurable objectives, select appropriate assessment and teaching strategies, and design effective instruction.

One of the most powerful contributions an ID can make is to design assessment instruments to measure actual learning outcomes (knowledge and skills) rather than participant satisfaction. For example, they can design the instruments to measure whether coaches have mastered the model, whether they can implement that model effectively, whether that results in learning (knowledge and skills) on the part of their coachees, and finally whether the coachees then in fact actually implement those skills in their own classrooms.

Activity Six: Analyzing Data and Reporting Results

The method of analysis depends on the evaluation questions and the standards selected. It is important to consider both the practical significance (how much impact the change represents) and statistical significance (whether the change is detectable by statistical measures). A lack of statistical significance may indicate that outcome measures were too ambitious or the desired behavioral change may take longer to emerge. Conversely, some nonsignificant findings may end up being useful for understanding or modifying the program. Interpreting results and drawing conclusions from program evaluations can be challenging. The involvement of stakeholders in reviewing findings and preliminary conclusions prior to writing a formal report is highly recommended.

KIRKPATRICK'S MODEL

Kirkpatrick's model has been widely used for conducting outcome evaluations of training programs.[7] This model supports the gathering of data to assess four "levels" of program outcomes (Table 11.4). There is also a fifth level to Kirkpatrick's model that focuses on return on investment (ROI). This fifth level was first posited by Phillips in his book *Return on Investment in Training and Performance Improvement Programs*.[8] However, this fifth level was not officially adopted by Kirkpatrick himself, who emphasized the need to conduct ROI calculations as an outcome measure for level 4.

Level 1: Learner Reaction or Satisfaction

This level evaluates how the participants who received training, in our case the coaches and coachees, feel about the training. It is important to measure participants' reactions so we understand how well the training was received and how to improve the training in the future. However, level 1 is insufficient on its own because it does not measure actual performance (whether the participants actually learned anything).

Level 1 data is important to collect, but it is also important to have higher level of evaluation to show that the program was not only popular but effective (and therefore, worth the investment).

Level 2: Learning

This level evaluates the actual learning (knowledge, skills, and attitudes) that results from the program. The learning objectives and related assessment items identified when the coaching session was planned help connect the changes in learning outcomes to the program rather than

TABLE 11.3   Common Challenges and Guidance for Data Collection (Activity 4)

Challenge	Explanation and Guidance
Assess in situ	Most of our assessment practices take place at the end of a workshop or session. Getting to the next level with coaching requires that assessment extend beyond the initial training we do (immediate posttest) to the actual environment—where the coaching itself occurs. This can take many forms. There are many ways to assess coaching posttraining, and the evaluation should use multiple measures for the purpose of triangulation. Options include delayed posttests, interviews with coaches and coachees, evaluation of coach/coachee diaries or logs, self-evaluation checklists around key features of the coaching process, and short answer responses to key questions done at regular intervals. The gold standard, however, is observation of coaches interacting with coachees in authentic sessions and using the same checklists and measures employed to assess outcomes in the training.
Training the trainer	The use of experts to deliver "the content" is one of the most powerful and unique aspects of coaching, yet it is potentially its greatest weakness. Although the focus of training coaches is on how to coach effectively (process rather than content), we sometimes also have expectations with regard to the content of what they coach. For example, we may intend for them to coach others on the implementation of a specific teaching strategy (e.g., active learning), which means that we care both about whether the coach is being a good coach and whether their coachees are learning how to implement the teaching strategy. To measure how well a coach coaches, we observe them coaching (how well they are implementing the coaching model itself). To measure how well they are promoting the teaching strategy (via the coaching process), we must also measure how well the coachees actually master the teaching strategy itself.
People, not tests	Learning outcomes always have a behavioral component—nobody just knows things, they do things with their knowledge—and it is that behavior that is the true measure of learning. Although paper tests of skills related to coaching are a necessary part of outcomes measurement, the sine qua non of measurement is the demonstration of coaching behavior. Roleplay is an example of both a good teaching and assessment strategy—pairing up with coaching trainees and having them coach the coach around predesigned scenarios that address the full range of coaching skill outcomes desired/planned might be helpful. This approach can serve as both practice and assessment during training and as follow-up testing later in situ.
Evaluating coaching in the environment	Coaching is optimally suited for Kirkpatrick's evaluation level 3: the environment. Coaches are intended to distribute expertise consistently and effectively throughout the organization. Tracking coaching activities routinely over time is important, such as • Counting sessions, if not actual session logs • Completion of evaluation forms for both coach and coachee two or three times per year • Asking coachees to maintain reflective journals of the coaching process • Conducting interviews with coach and coachee dyads for triangulation and setting a schedule so that all coaches are interviewed once per year in the beginning • Most importantly, using this data both for program reporting (outcomes) *and* for modifying the program itself (process) to maintain high-quality implementation

to environmental influences. These learning outcomes are commonly measured before and after the training. Although evaluations that assess levels 1 and 2 are often sufficient for evaluating the training itself, they are not sufficient to answer

questions about the effects of the intervention outside the confines of the intervention itself (e.g., transfer of learning to the workplace). Unless we are able to show that coaches and coachees truly mastered the intended objectives, there

TABLE 11.4 Kirkpatrick's Evaluation Model		
Levels	**Key Features**	**Cautions and Caveats**
Level 1: Reaction/ satisfaction	• Evaluates how participants *perceive* the training	• Measures *perception,* not *learning*
Level 2: Learning	• Evaluates actual *learning*	• Measured before and after training
Level 3: Behavior	• Whether what was *learned* (level 2) actually *transfers* to the workplace • Focus is on behavioral changes • Observations/interviews with employees/supervisors are common	• May take weeks or months to manifest/assess • Environmental pressures may prevent change
Level 4: Results	• Impact of changed behavior on the organization	• Requires significant resources/long-term commitment • Best reserved for mission-critical outcomes and long-term programs

is no way to tell the difference between great teachers who did not learn from the program and poor teachers who did.

Level 3: Behavior

This level evaluates whether what participants learned (e.g., changes, in knowledge, skills, and attitudes measured at level 2) actually transfers beyond the intervention to the workplace. We need to be aware that change in behavior is a longer-term activity, and it might take several weeks or months after the initial training to demonstrate accurate results. One of the best ways to measure behavior is to conduct observations and interviews over time and to compare them to how the trainees have applied the information they received compared with a preferred standard. Another area to consider is to what extent the conditions of the environment are favorable to any behavior changes. As such, level 3 would require that we would be able to show how well coaches' knowledge and skills translated to on-the-job behavior. Put another way, just because coaches know what to do does not mean they will choose to do it or that the environment will allow them to do it.

Level 3 is hard to achieve consistently as it requires the resources to observe and evaluate all coaches and coachees at least once. It is well worth the investment early on in the program, however, as it is the most powerful form of evidence that a program is working. It would be important to do this at least once in the first year for the coaches and the coachees if there is an expected, observable behavioral outcome. After the first year, continued positive results from level 2 evaluation combined with this evidence from the first year may suffice if resources cannot be committed over the long term. If not always possible, selecting a random or

stratified sample of coaches and coachees to observe can save time and resources while still providing some evidence for level 3.

Level 4: Results

This level is the hardest to achieve and requires the most resources. That's because this level refers to the impact of the program (levels 1, 2, and 3) on the bottom line of the organization. Thus it should be reserved for the most mission-critical outcomes of programs that are expected to have a widespread effect and to continue over significant periods of time (years, not weeks). Measuring these results can be costly and time-consuming. The biggest challenge is selecting those results or outcomes that are most closely linked to the program and finding effective ways to measure them over the long term. Some examples include the effect on patient outcomes, cost savings and reduced waste across the system, increased retention or morale, and higher quality ratings. For a coaching program, this would likely require tracking things longitudinally, such as student retention rates, graduation rates, honors, faculty retention, time-to-tenure and promotion, publication rates, and education-related grant writing, and correlate those with time and money saved, public reputation, etc. In truth, the institution would need to be almost as responsible for this level of assessment, and the resources needed to do this would not likely be justified by a coaching program.

RETURN ON INVESTMENT

The real value of conducting an evaluation lies in being able to use the results (in this case, level 4) to calculate ROI.

TABLE 11.5 **Primary Steps Involved in Calculating Return on Investment (ROI)**
1. Use control groups, if possible, and comparison groups if not.
2. Allow enough time for results to be achieved and measurable.
3. Determine the direct and indirect costs of the training (time, salary, materials, lost productivity).
4. Measure outcomes data before, during, and after the training.
5. Measure the performance increase relative to prior performance.
6. Translate the performance increase into a dollar value benefit (e.g., saved time is multiplied by salary for each person affected).
7. Subtract the dollar value benefit from the cost of training.
8. Use the result to calculate the ROI.

However, ROI cannot be calculated meaningfully if data are missing, data are of poor quality (e.g., using likability ratings or self-report for learning outcomes), or there are no high-quality standards of performance. Like level 4, ROI itself requires significant investment. It is best to establish the relative importance of the program to the organization up front and to identify the resources and commitment from the administration that will allow an ROI analysis to be conducted. Table 11.5 presents some of the primary steps outlined by Phillips[4] to calculate ROI.

FINAL THOUGHTS ON KIRKPATRICK'S MODEL

Although Kirkpatrick's model is popular and widely used, there are several considerations that need to be taken into account when using it. Collecting data for levels 3 and 4 can be an expensive and time-consuming activity, especially if the institution doesn't have dedicated personnel or does not have the systems in place to collect these types

of data regularly. Depending on the scale of the intervention and the number of other ongoing evaluations, level 3 could be feasibly done by a small staff over time. However, level 4 almost certainly requires multiple, dedicated staff and cooperation. Also, institutions continuously change, and separating out the program effects from the multitude of other factors is challenging under the best of circumstances.

This does not mean we should abandon those levels. Even when resources are limited, there is always a way to evaluate levels 3 and 4. Wedman and Tessmer's Layers of Necessity model[5] suggests that constraints should be used to adjust, not eliminate, what is done at a stage of a process (e.g., evaluation). Ron Zemke makes the same point about needs assessment—there is always time to do something.[9] If the behavior of everyone who has been coached cannot be observed (level 3), taking a random sample or a purposive sample of the most typical participants can be done. If a sample of that many people can't be observed, choosing one to observe and surveying the others can be an alternative. Each option is less robust than the one before, but anything is better than nothing. It is important to be clear about how representative and reliable the data are.

SUMMARY

Evaluations can provide process data on the successes and challenges of early implementation or, for more mature programs, can provide outcome data on program participants. The information obtained can help target program resources in the most cost-efficient way. The key is to understand what questions we want to answer, adopt an appropriate model with which we are familiar, conduct evaluation concurrently with program design if possible, and measure how well the program is being implemented (process) as well as its impact on the organization (outcomes or goals). Although program evaluations may seem complicated, expensive, or even overwhelming, they can be deployed effectively even by nonevaluation experts by determining the purpose of the evaluation, focusing on the six common evaluation activities, and considering the level of the evaluation we wish to achieve.

TAKE-HOME POINTS

1. Program evaluation depends on what we and other stakeholders want to learn; the clearer we are about our goals and questions we want answered, the more effective we will be.

2. Evaluation and intervention planning should occur concurrently for best results.
3. Evaluation should begin before, and continue after, the launch of the intervention itself.

4. Defining success criteria and ensuring stakeholders' participation before selecting evaluation measures is important.
5. Tracking benefits well after the coaching training is over, including Kirkpatrick's level 3 (transfer of the intervention to the workplace), level 4 (impact on the organization itself), and ROI should be considered.
6. Evaluation plans must be adjusted to reflect institutional resources. Failure to be realistic leads to a "stuck" evaluation (inability to reach the level it is designed for) or one that produces unreliable data.
7. Evaluation of the program should include evaluation of the evaluation itself to make sure it reflects the design of the program as it is proceeding.

QUESTIONS FOR FURTHER THOUGHT

1. As you reflect on your own coaching program, what can you conclude from your evaluation efforts? Are your outcomes and questions representative of what you want to know?
2. What are the standards that you use to determine whether your program is effective? Do you have all the data and processes you need to be able to answer those questions?
3. Is your coaching program effective? For whom? Under what circumstances? Which components of your coaching program are more or least effective?
4. How do the results of your evaluation compare in whole or in part with findings from similar coaching programs implemented elsewhere?
5. What changes can be made to your coaching program (and your evaluation processes) in terms of content (goals/objectives), activities, and processes to expand its scope and effectiveness?

ANNOTATED BIBLIOGRAPHY

Kirkpatrick D. Revisiting Kirkpatrick's four-level model. *Training Dev*. 1996;50:54–58.
   This is an updated review of Kirkpatrick's model of education, with particular focus on training programs and current business environments (e.g., the need for return on investment for training programs).
Phillips JJ. *Return on Investment in Training and Performance Improvement Programs*, 2nd edition. London: Routledge; 2011.
   This is an excellent treatise on conducting return on investment (ROI) assessments for training programs. Although not focused on coaching specifically, the approach is applicable, and this has been considered a definitive text on the theory and practice of conducting ROI.

REFERENCES

1. McGovern J, Lindemann M, Vergara MA, Murphy S, Barker L, Warrenfeltz R. Maximizing the impact of executive coaching: behavioral change, organizational outcomes and return on investment. *J People and Organ Transition. Manchester Rev.* 2001;6(1):1–9.
2. Fillery-Travis A, Lane D. Does coaching work or are we asking the wrong question? *Int Coach Psychol Rev*. 2006(1):23–36.
3. ACGME. Accreditation council for graduate medical education: glossary of terms. Accreditation Council for Graduate Medical Education. April 15, 2020. http://www.acgme.org/acWebsitte/about/ab_ACGMEglossary.pdf. Accessed August 3, 2021.
4. Phillips JJ. *Return on Investment in Training and Performance Improvement Programs*. 2nd ed.: Butterworth Heinemann Publishers; 1997.
5. Frye AW, Hemmer PA. Program evaluation models and related theories: AMEE Guide No. 67. *Med Teach*. 2012:68.
6. Leonard-Cross E. Developmental coaching: business benefit: fact or fad? An evaluative study to explore the impact of coaching in the workplace. *Int Coaching Psychol Rev*. 2010;5(1):36–47.
7. Kirkpatrick D. Revisiting Kirkpatrick's four-level model. *Training Dev*. 1996;50(1):54–58.
8. Phillips JJ. *Return on Investment in Training and Performance Improvement Programs*. 2nd ed. London: Routledge; 2011.
9. Zemke R. How to do a needs assessment when you think you don't have time. *Training*. 1998;35(3):38.

The Current and Future State of Coaching in Medical Education

Jean E. Klig, Michael A. Haight, and Michele A. Favreau

LEARNING OBJECTIVES

1. Identify areas where coaching has demonstrated the greatest impact for performance improvement.
2. Describe coaching outcomes and future research directions.
3. Synthesize the most effective components of multidisciplinary coaching frameworks.
4. Establish cost-value outcomes for coaching.

CHAPTER OUTLINE

CHAPTER SUMMARY

This chapter examines the current best evidence on the impact of coaching and essential outcomes that support its expanded use in medical education and identifies gaps that can be addressed through further research. We include evidence from nonmedical disciplines to contextualize opportunities for progress and to propose future avenues for research that can advance coaching practices and applications in medicine. Our discussion highlights how a shared understanding of coaching definitions, applications, and practices is necessary to be able to consistently measure the effectiveness of coaching in medical education. We explore ways to establish the value of coaching in medical education via return on investment concepts and metrics and describe its implications for future research. Finally, we delineate a trajectory for future coaching research in medical education.

INTRODUCTION

What can coaching add to medical education and what justifies its cost? These questions inevitably arise with novel approaches to teaching and learning, and the business literature already provides helpful evidence for the value of coaching. To promulgate the use of coaching in medical education, we must consider why, how, when, and where it can add value to existing pedagogical approaches. The current literature provides data on the early impact of coaching that can serve as a roadmap for future research to elucidate its broader effects, build on existing frameworks and outcomes, and justify its value within medical education. This chapter examines current evidence on coaching in medical education and considers the key practice elements and outcome metrics that can shape future research. We then leverage these sections with an evaluation of return on investment (ROI) considerations that are essential to successfully advance the use of coaching within medical education research and practice. By reviewing the research and gaps therein, we suggest a blueprint for future coaching education research.

COACHING IMPACT IN MEDICAL EDUCATION

Coaching offers a versatile strategy to engage learners and promote learning, which is reflected in the coaching applications introduced in medical education since 2010 to address goals from skill performance to well-being.[1] Initial research demonstrates the early impact of coaching and establishes its potential for future applications. Promising early progress on validity evidence for instruments to assess coaching in medical education is supported by outcomes evidence from other disciplines.[2] Two key questions frame a future research agenda for coaching in medical education: What areas of medical education do we know improve the most with coaching, and what aspects of research on coaching effectiveness from other disciplines can we apply to medicine?

Coaching Evidence in Medical Education

The early literature demonstrating the effects of coaching in medical education primarily encompasses four topic areas: clinical procedural skills; academics and/or professional identity formation; feedback; and wellness. Overall, the current evidence uses research outcomes that include feasibility of coaching as an educational strategy, learner reactions, and test performance. These outcomes reflect lower tier or early progress based on Kirkpatrick's model yet provide an important foundation for further research.

Current research evidence most supports the effects of coaching to improve surgical procedure skills.[3,4] Beyond direct coaching in the operating room, a novel application of video-based coaching after a surgical procedure demonstrates its effect on learning, with an increase in teaching points per unit time, statistically significant greater resident initiative to direct their education, and more coach-initiated questions to promote critical thinking and set learning goals.[5] Further studies support the value and feasibility of coaching-enabled videotape review and/or simulation to advance the development of surgical procedural skills. These studies and clinical skills data[6] provide an impetus for broader research on the applications of coaching in skills teaching across medicine.

The implementation of coaching for academic development and/or professional identity formation is highlighted by the current literature as a promising avenue for learner engagement and competency development. Research studies on academic coaching provide data that

---

Vignette 1

Dr. Evidence is a clinical clerkship director who plans to introduce coaching to her rotation. Coaching will be a completely new experience for the students and one that seems worthwhile to increase their engagement in clinical learning. She decides to focus on using coaching for feedback on both clinical performance and procedures. After a review of the current literature for guidance, she decides to pilot the R2C2 model as a framework that preceptors can use to provide feedback after clinical encounters during the clerkship. She also decides to use coached video-based review as an approach to feedback on procedures. There is still some time for further planning before the new changes to the clerkship will be launched.

Thought Questions

1. How can Dr. Evidence introduce the role of coaching to the faculty preceptors based on her plan?
2. What outcomes can Dr. Evidence use to evaluate the use of coached video-based review with her students?

---

identifies key factors for successful coaching experiences[1,7] and demonstrate a positive impact on clinical learning and development for medical students and residents. One study also shows a beneficial effect of coaching in the early identification of at-risk students, thereby facilitating prompt remediation for these students.[7] More limited evidence suggests that coaching may improve reflective practice[8] that is pivotal to academic development and can support professional identity formation.[9] Further research is needed to clarify how coaching can be systematically applied for academic development and professional identity formation across the competency continuum and what coaching practices and programs are most impactful to learner success.

Feedback is an essential part of the learning process, and it is more effectively sustained through coaching. The R2C2 model for feedback[10] delineates a four-part process that includes coaching as its final step. In this model, coaching promotes the opportunity for a conversation in which the learner can assess and integrate feedback. The R2C2 model thus adds yet another dimension to the impact of coaching in medical education. Although the current data for the R2C2 model addresses graduate medical education alone, its overall framework is applicable to medical student education and remains a promising area for future research. Existing data showing the positive effect of coaching medical students to receive feedback[11] supports an expanded role for coaching in feedback conversations to enhance learning.

Psychological wellness is increasingly recognized as an important factor to improve learner engagement and optimize learning. Initial studies on wellness coaching have examined its impact on medical student and resident progress. Smaller scale studies involving medical students demonstrate progress from coaching in terms of adaptability and proactive learning on a clerkship[12] and increases in self-efficacy for overall stress management.[13] Similarly, the use of the principles of positive psychology for coaching toward wellness in professional development is demonstrated to produce lower rates of burnout in residents.[14] Future research may address how coaching can consistently and effectively augment trainee wellness and how it can be integrated into overall academic coaching.

The overall effect of coaching in medical education may be optimally viewed in the context of the range of learning activities and interactions that physician trainees experience, where different time-variable approaches to coaching might suit different learning situations. Landreville et al. propose a bilevel coaching model for medical education with "coaching in the moment" (CiM) and "coaching over time" (CoT) approaches.[15] CiM occurs in the clinical environment and necessitates a more directive coaching approach during which the coach provides actionable and immediate feedback. CoT primarily occurs outside of the clinical environment and entails a longitudinal, collaborative coaching approach in which the coach and learner review performance data, engage in bidirectional feedback, and cocreate suggestions for improvement. This model provides an essential distinction between two key approaches to coaching in medical education that can be expanded through future research in coaching applications. Moreover, each approach warrants further study to determine effective measurements, appropriate outcomes, and impact across the spectrum of coaching in medical education.

Coaching Evidence Beyond Medical Education

Coaching has been well-known to the business world for decades, and it has been an integral part of sports and music for even longer. Each of these disciplines requires a unique focus on individual performance as the basis for coaching, which can also have an effect at a team or organizational level. The impact of coaching in music or sports can be viewed as more linear, as the goal of a specific performance or event can be judged via metrics such as quality, technique, audience response, or "winning." Coaching in both music and sports demonstrates the high yield of a coach-coachee dyad to enhance individual performance. This is perhaps most recognizable in sports as coaching toward a "personal best," with the coach-athlete relationship at the

Vignette 2

Dr. Westin is the program director for a medium-sized family medicine program at an academic health center. A year ago, she started an informal coaching program for residents to support performance improvement and wellness. Faculty volunteer coaches and residents alike were pleased with the program and anecdotally reported positive outcomes. Dr. Westin would now like to formalize the coaching program and is developing a coaching program proposal for her department chair. Dr. Westin is working with her faculty team to develop coaching outcomes for her new coaching program. The team seems to be struggling to create outcomes other than those that indicate "satisfaction."

Thought Questions

1. How might Dr. Westin best use the anecdotal data from her informal coaching program to create measurable outcomes for her new coaching program?
2. What types of evidence can Dr. Westin use to help her evaluate the effectiveness of her proposed coaching program?

heart of the success.[3] A parallel in the business world is executive coaching, where individual performance gains can have a significant impact on organizational gains and financial yield.[16] Data on the effect of coaching in business continues to introduce metrics to sufficiently capture the financial yield that can better calibrate its use.[16,17] However, research from the business literature also emphasizes the value of coaching for individual performance to promote organizational success at levels beyond specific financial gain. "Human capital, the idea that people represent more than tangible assets and are in fact organizational investors in a knowledge economy rather than organizational costs, has begun to change the way we think about such questions as *Did coaching help the business?*"[17] Evidence on the impact of coaching reaches beyond business, music, and sports to include higher education, where it is highlighted as "a powerful tool for learning and personal growth" that benefits students, teachers, educational leaders, and establishments.[18] Viewed as a whole, these provide an auspicious view of the impact that coaching can have toward progress in medical education that is learner-centered and ultimately cost-effective compared with traditional approaches. Future research is needed to elucidate the broader applications of coaching in medical education and to define outcomes that optimally demonstrate its multifaceted impact on teaching and learning.

MEASURING COACHING EFFECTIVENESS

It is essential to measure the effectiveness of coaching in order to better define the role and value of coaching in medical education. However, because of the complex nature of coaching, valid and reliable coaching effectiveness studies have proven elusive in the literature. Although there are numerous cross-disciplinary coaching studies on coaching effectiveness, many of these rely on arbitrary, practitioner-generated evaluation approaches that are not uniform.[19,20] In addition, many coaching studies tend to use retrospective, self-report methods to determine coaching effectiveness. These types of studies lend themselves to subjective judgments about coaching effectiveness.[19,20] This has led to a small body of coaching effectiveness research that has produced varied results. The lack of a systematic approach to evaluating the effectiveness of coaching has engendered skepticism by many, especially given the high costs associated with coaching.[21,22] Research that objectifies and quantifies coaching is quite limited and continues to pose challenges for researchers. This is an area of great opportunity for ongoing studies.

A framework for evaluating the value of coaching exists as ROI in the business literature.[23] However, the idiosyncratic nature of ROI is not without its challenges, and researchers recommend that ROI should be triangulated with other data points for a more comprehensive interpretation of coaching effectiveness.[19,20] The Coaching Effectiveness Survey (CES), developed by the Institute for Executive Coaching and Leadership (IECL), is a reliable measure of the effectiveness of coaching engagements, but the authors caution that survey data is subjective and not all relevant components of the coaching process can be measured.[24] As is the same with most coaching effectiveness surveys, the CES only measures outcomes at the conclusion of coaching, not at specified intervals across the coaching experience, so it is difficult to determine incremental progress across time. There is a need for more research to measure coaching outcomes across designated periods of time, rather than merely as a single, end-of-program outcome. Additionally, in order to better determine coaching outcomes and effectiveness, coaching studies need to contextualize coaching within an organization to capture the complexities of its overall impact.[20]

Preliminary data based on coaching outcomes across disciplines indicate that coaching is an effective intervention.[19,20,24] Common coaching outcomes include performance improvement, skill development, increased coping strategies, improved work attitudes, goal-directed self-regulation, self-efficacy, self-awareness, and well-being.[19,20,24] Coaching outcomes can occur at an individual or organizational level. However, most coaching studies have focused their results on individual, rather than organizational, outcomes.[19,20] In order to better determine coaching outcomes and effectiveness, coaching studies need to contextualize coaching within an organization to capture its overall impact on both the individual and the organization.[19,20] Evers et al. and Moen et al. posit that coaching positively affects goal-attainment expectancy and goal progression and commitment.[25,26] Kampa-Kokesh reports that there is evidence to support coaching as an effective intervention for improving performance and facilitating behavioral change.[27] Grant et al. showed that coaching enhanced goal achievement, resilience, and workplace well-being and demonstrated that coaching had a positive impact on coping and self-regulation.[28] Duijits et al. noted an increase in well-being and life satisfaction for employees working in medical, health, and educational organizations as the result of coaching.[29] Researchers caution though that validating these types of coaching outcomes in the coaching literature can be challenging because of the heterogeneity of coaching research frameworks.[19,20]

Studies that examined the impact of the number of coaching sessions on coaching outcomes showed that a greater number of sessions did not necessarily produce greater positive effects. In fact, for some outcomes, an increased number of sessions produced a potentially negative effect.[19,20] For example, positive results from coaching correlated with fewer sessions for performance improvement, skill development, and work attitudes. This might be attributed to the type of coaching intervention or the scope of the issue addressed by coaching.[20]

Coaching effectiveness research shows that, because coaching is fluid and dynamic, it behaves as a "complex adaptive system."[30,31] Grover and Fuhrnam describe this complexity by noting that there are most likely a number of factors and characteristics that potentially interact with one another to create success through the complex interactions of coaching.[18] They investigate "distal" outcomes and describe "moderators" and "mediators" of outcomes in an effort to identify relevant factors that affect coaching outcomes. They suggest that coachee, coach, and the relationship between them are primary "mediators" or "moderators" that exist "between variables" to drive the coaching experience and engender success.[19,20] Sonesh et al.[32] further contend that coaching more strongly affects "relationship outcomes" rather than "goal-attainment outcomes."[31] Therefore, specific coachee and coach characteristics and their effect on the coaching relationship warrant further study.[19,20,33]

Studying coaching effectiveness then is a nascent field that would benefit from establishing a uniform theoretical framework that encapsulates the inherent complexities of the entire coaching process. Such a framework would help create a standardized foundation for more homogeneity in the design of future coaching effectiveness studies and the generalization of coaching outcomes.

RETURN ON INVESTMENT FOR COACHING IN MEDICAL EDUCATION

Over the past two decades, coaching research in business has focused on ROI. Coaching in the business setting evolved from use as a remedial action into a strategy for developing maximal business benefit. Corporations use ROI to show a return on their learning, development, and performance improvement costs for their leadership and organization.

The Manchester Review Study is the most frequently cited work that has explored coaching ROI.[34] This seminal work involved studies of senior-level executives at Fortune 1000 companies who received developmental coaching and were asked to quantify the impact of coaching on their business. Researchers calculated ROI and made adjustments to isolate the effects of the coaching. Results demonstrated that the average ROI was five times the initial investment. Further research in medical education is necessary to determine how to replicate these outcomes across the spectrum of medical education.

ROI can be measured with both soft and hard data. The goal of coaching is to improve performance and change behavior with developmental shifts over time. Laske proposed that behavior change takes time and time has a cost.[35] Because behavior change is measurable, an ROI can be generated by measuring both time and behavioral change.

There is an ongoing debate about using ROI as an effective method to evaluate coaching.[36] De Meuse et al. question its usefulness and veracity due to the lack of consensus and its lack of dimensionality.[37] Theeboom et al. note that coaching is effective in individual level outcomes such as performance skills, well-being, and coping.[20] However, translating those outcome categories into a financial tool is exceedingly difficult. Grant argues that ROI is a poor measure of coaching success because of the variability of metric meaning and excessive focus on financial outcomes.[38] He instead advocates for measurement of well-being and engagement rather than financial change. Thus adequately measuring ROI for coaching necessitates triangulation of data from multiple different sources to effectively determine its impact.

Although medical educators recognize the need to quantify the value of coaching to justify its inclusion in their medical education curricula, there is not a robust body of literature to help guide these efforts. Ongoing, high-quality research on the ROI in medical education is essential to identify evidence-based applications of ROI

Vignette 3

Dr. North is the chair of a large, academic pediatric department. She has decided to start a department-wide coaching program for both the trainees and faculty. Dr. North is anxious to move forward with establishing the coaching program, but her administrator is concerned about the costs and the potential impact this program might have on faculty productivity. The administrator has requested a financial proposal from Dr. North.

Thought Questions

1. How might Dr. North apply ROI assessment methods to justify her coaching program?
2. What are the limitations to existing ROI metrics?

---

in medical education, optimize the outcomes of coaching, and maximize the costs of coaching programs.[39]

DIRECTIONS FOR FUTURE RESEARCH

Coaching in medical education has demonstrated effectiveness as a clinical tool for the development of procedural skills. Preliminary data also suggest that coaching can be beneficial as a tool to support learner receptivity to feedback and to promote learner wellness. These positive outcomes have demonstrated enhanced learner performance. Although coaching can be used to address academic development and professional identity formation, there remains insufficient research data to determine whether coaching significantly affects the academic and professional development of physicians. Current models of coaching in medical education suggest the application of different coaching timeframes for different learning environments, necessitating the need for further research on the overall outcomes and impact for each of these models. Future coaching studies should likewise focus on the individual characteristics of the coach and coachee and how these affect the overall coaching experience in order to determine their potential impact on promoting academic and professional development.

Lack of a universally accepted definition of coaching in medical education limits the ability to measure coaching effectiveness. The ubiquitous use of less rigorous research methods such as self-report and coach-generated collection makes it difficult to generalize coaching outcomes and affect the reliability and validity of coaching research studies. Establishing a shared framework for the concept of coaching in medical education would serve to produce more targeted research with more reliable outcomes.

Published studies that specifically address ROI for coaching in medical education are not yet present in the medical education literature. However, the business literature has provided a model for ROI studies that might be useful in determining coaching "value" in medical education. Research that focuses on coaching value as ROI might help provide justification for developing coaching programs across the continuum of medical education.

As coaching evolves to be more ubiquitous in medical education, so too must coaching research evolve to delineate the validity, reliability, and value of coaching as an educational tool. The limited nature of the coaching literature in medical education can and should serve as an opportunity and impetus for all medical educators to study coaching programs in their own learning environments. As a community of medical educational researchers, we can begin to fill in the research gaps and produce strong evidence for the development of coaching programs across the spectrum of medical education. Only through our collective efforts can we fully realize the utility, impact, and value of coaching in medical education. We hope this book will provide the foundation to adapt common coaching definitions, frameworks, and competencies so we can validate the value of coaching in medical education, including successfully integrating competency-based medical education and producing master adaptive leaners.

TAKE-HOME POINTS

1. Coaching has been demonstrated to improve surgical procedure skills, with evidence for academic coaching, coaching for feedback, and wellness coaching gaining in scope and proven outcomes across the continuum of medical education.

2. The success of coaching in business, sports, music, and higher education demonstrates its value as a learner-driven process of performance improvement and achievement of personal goals.

3. Coaching effectiveness research would benefit from a universal theoretical coaching framework to better design coaching studies and measure coaching effectiveness.

4. Preliminary cross-disciplinary data indicate that coaching has a positive impact on skill development, performance improvement, behavioral change, life satisfaction, and well-being. There is a need to conduct more research to better understand the application of these outcomes in medical education.

5. ROI can be useful to assess the value of coaching but should not be used as a measurement in isolation.

ANNOTATED BIBLIOGRAPHY

Landreville J, Cheung W, Frank J, Richardson, D. A definition for coaching in medical education. *Can Med Educ J.* 2019;10(4):e109–e110.
Proposes time-variable models (coaching in the moment and coaching over time) for coaching across different learning environments in medical education.

Lovell B. What do we know about coaching in medical education? A literature review. *Med Educ.* 2018;52(4):376–390.
A critical review of the research literature on coaching in medical education that is important to our understanding of the gaps in what is currently known.

McGovern J, Lindermann M, Vergara M, et al. Maximizing the impact of executive coaching: Behavioral change, organizational outcomes and return on investment. *Manch Rev (Bala Cynwyd Pa).* 2001;6(1):1–9.
Seminal study on ROI for executive coaching in business. Contains in-depth analyses of the multiple dimensions involved in coaching and describes how different aspects of coaching interface to create ROI.

Theeboom T. Beersma B, van Vianen EM. Does coaching work? A meta-analysis on the effects of coaching on individual level outcomes in an organizational context. *J Posit Psychol.* 2013;9(1):1–18.

A scoping review of cross-disciplinary educational coaching models. Includes critical analyses of coaching methods, metrics, outcomes, and impacts.

REFERENCES

1. Wolff M, Morgan H, Hammoud M, Ross PT. Academic coaching: Insights from the medical student's perspective. *Med Teach.* 2019;42(2):172–177.
2. Carney PA, Bonura EM, Kraakevik JA, Juve AM, Kahl LE, Deiorio NM. Measuring coaching in undergraduate medical education: the development and psychometric validation of new instruments. *J Gen Intern Med.* 2019; 34(5):677–683.
3. Lovell B. What do we know about coaching in medical education? A literature review. *Med Educ.* 2018;52(4):376–390. doi:10.1111/medu.13482.
4. Gagnon LH, Abbasi N. Systematic review of randomized controlled trials on the role of coaching in surgery to improve learner outcomes. *Am J Surg.* 2018;216(1):140–146.
5. Hu YY, Mazer LM, Yule SJ, et al. Complementing operating room teaching with video-based coaching. *JAMA Surgery.* 2017;152(4):318–325.
6. Rassbach CE, Blankenburg R. A novel pediatric residency coaching program: Outcomes after one year. *Acad Med.* 2017;93(3):430–434.

7. Régo P, Peterson R, Callaway L, et al. Using a structured clinical coaching program to improve clinical skills training and assessment, as well as teachers' and students' satisfaction. *Med Teach*. 2009;31(12):586–595.

8. Könings KD, van Berlo J, Koopmans R, et al. Using a Smartphone App and Coaching Group Sessions to Promote Residents' Reflection in the Workplace. *Acad Med*. 2016;91(3):365–370.

9. de Lasson L, Just E, Stegeager N, Malling B. Professional identity formation in the transition from medical school to working life: A qualitative study of group-coaching courses for junior doctors. *BMC Med Educ*. 2016;16(1).

10. Sargeant J, Armson H, Driessen E, et al. Evidence-Informed Facilitated Feedback: The R2C2 Feedback Model. *MedEdPORTAL*. 2016;12(1) mep2374-8265.10387.

11. Bing-You RG, Bertsch T, Thompson JA. Coaching medical students in receiving effective feedback. *Teach Learn Med*. 1998;10(4):228–231.

12. Guseh SH, Chen XP, Johnson NR. Can enriching emotional intelligence improve medical students' proactivity and adaptability during OB/GYN clerkships? *Int J Med Educ*. 2015;6:208–212.

13. Cameron D, Dromerick LJ, Ahn J, Dromerick AW. Executive/life coaching for first year medical students: A prospective study. *BMC Med Educ*. 2019;19(1).

14. Palamara K, Kauffman C, Chang Y, et al. professional development coaching for residents: results of a 3-year positive psychology coaching intervention. *J Gen Intern Med*. 2018;33(11):1842–1844.

15. Landreville J, Cheung W, Frank J, Richardson D. A definition for coaching in medical education. *Can Med Educ J*. 2019;10(4):e109–e110.

16. Levenson A. Measuring and maximizing the business impact of executive coaching. *Consult Psychol J Pract Res*. 2009;61(2):103–121.

17. Schlosser B, Steinbrenner D, Kumata E, Hunt J. The coaching impact study: measuring the value of executive coaching with commentary. *International Journal of Coaching in Organizations*. 2007;5(1):140–161.

18. Capstick MK, Harrell-Williams LM, Cockrum CD, West SL. Exploring the effectiveness of academic coaching for academically at-risk college students. *Innov High Educ*. 2019;44(3):219–231.

19. Grover S, Furnham A. Coaching as a developmental intervention in organizations: A systematic review of its effectiveness and mechanisms underlying it. *PLoS ONE*. 2016;11(7):e0159137.

20. Theeboom T, Beersma B, van Vianen EM. Does coaching work? A meta-analysis on the effects of coaching on individual level outcomes in an organizational context. *J Posit Psychol*. 2013;9(1):1–18.

21. Bozer G, Sarros JC. Examining the effectiveness of executive coaching on coaches' performance in the Israeli context. *Int J Evid Based Coach Mentor*. 2012;10:14–32.

22. Bono JE, Purvanova RK, Towler A, Peterson DB. A survey of executive coaching practices. *Pers Psychol*. 2012;62:361–404.

23. Phillips JJ. Measuring the ROI of a coaching intervention. Part 2. *Performance Improvement*. 2007;46(10):10–23.

24. Tooth J-A, Nielsen S, Armstrong H. Coaching effectiveness survey instruments: taking stock of measuring the immeasurable. *Coaching: An International Journal of Theory, Research & Practice*. 2013;6(2):137–151.

25. Evers WJ, Brouwer A, Tomic W. A quasi-experimental study on management coaching effectiveness. *Consult Psychol J Pract Res*. 2006;58:174–182.

26. Moen F, Skaalvik E. The effect from coaching on performance psychology. *Int J Evid Based Coach Ment*. 2009;7:1–49.

27. Kampa-Kokesch S, Anderson MZ. Executive coaching: A comprehensive review of the literature. *Consult Psychol J Pract Res*. 2001;53:205–228.

28. Grant AM, Curtayne L, Burton G. Executive coaching enhances goal attainment, resilience and workplace well being: A randomised controlled study. *J Posit Psychol*. 2009;4:396–407.

29. Duijts SFA, Kant IP, van den Brandt PAP, Swaen GMH. Effectiveness of a preventive coaching intervention for employees at risk for sickness absence due to psychosocial health complaints: Results of a randomized controlled trial. *J Occup Environ Med*. 2008;50:765–776.

30. Jones R, Brown D. The mentoring relationship as a complex adaptive system: Finding a model for our experience. *Mentor Tutoring*. 2011;9(4):401–418.

31. Holland JH. Studying complex adaptive systems. *J Syst Sci Complex*. 2006:1–8 19d.

32. Sonesh SC, Coultas CW, Lacerenza CN, et al. The power of coaching: a meta-analytic investigation. *Coaching: An International Journal of Theory, Research and Practice*. 2015;8(2):73–95.

33. Bozer G, Joo B-K, Joseph SC. Executive coaching: Does coach-coachee matching based on similarity really matter? *Consult Psychol J Pract Res*. 2015;67:218–233.

34. McGovern J, Lindermann M, Vergara M, et al. Maximizing the impact of executive coaching: Behavioral change, organizational outcomes and return on investment. *The Manchester Review*. 2001;6(1):1–9.

35. Laske O. Can evidence based coaching increase ROI? *Int J Evid Based Coach Mentor*. 2004;2(2):1–12.

36. Passmore J, Gibbes C. The state of executive coaching research: What does the current literature tell us and what's the next for coaching research. *Int Coach Psychol Rev*. 2007;2(2):116–128.

37. De Meuse K, Dai G, Lee R. Evaluating the effectiveness of executive coaching: beyond ROI. *Coaching: An International Journal of Theory, Practice and Research*. 2009;2(2):117–134.

38. Grant AM. ROI is a poor measure of coaching success: Towards a more holistic approach using a well-being and engagement framework. *Coaching: An International Journal of Theory, Research and Practice*. 2012;5(2):74–85.

39. Passmore J, Fillery-Travis A. A critical review of executive coaching research: a decade of progress and what's to come. *Coaching: An International Journal of Theory, Research and Practice*. 2011;4(2):70–88.

A

acceptance and commitment therapy Applied by coaches in leadership and well-being. It is also described as emotional agility.

advising Provides learners with expert answers to their questions. Not to be confused with coaching or mentoring.

appreciative inquiry Uses a strengths-based approach to engage learners in identifying their strengths and postulating how those strengths can be used to achieve desired outcomes.

autonomy Self-determination.

B

behavioral psychology Systematic approach to understanding the behavior of humans and other animals that assumes behavior is either a reflex evoked by the pairing of certain antecedent stimuli in the environment or a consequence of that individual's history.

bias An inclination of temperament or outlook. A personal and sometimes unreasoned judgment. Can be helpful or harmful. A systematic departure from the truth due to design or measurement characteristics.

Bloom's taxonomy Set of three hierarchical models used to classify educational learning objectives into levels of complexity and specificity.

burnout State of emotional, physical, and mental exhaustion caused by excessive and prolonged stress.

C

change management models Describe and simplify a process in a way everyone can understand. Several models are available.

character strengths Positive parts of personality that impact thinking, feelings, and behavior.

clinical performance examinations (CPXs) A practical test of general clinical knowledge.

coachee A person being coached.

coaching A coach helps a learner review and understand their assessments, identify needs and goals, and create a plan to move toward goals. A coach helps the learner be accountable, to improve self-monitoring, and to realize full potential. Not to be confused with advising or mentoring.

Coaching in Medicine model Based on the principles of growth mindset, reflective practice, self-determination theory, lifelong learning, and goal setting.

coaching psychology A branch of psychology concerned with the systematic application of the behavioral science of psychology to the enhancement of life experience, work performance, and well-being for individuals, groups, and organizations.

cognitive load theory Refers to the number of resources available in a learner's working memory at a given time.

community of practice A group of people who share a concern or a passion for something they do and learn how to do it better as they interact regularly.

competency-based medical education An outcomes-based approach to the design, implementation, and evaluation of education programs and the assessment of learners, using competencies or observable abilities. The goal is to ensure all learners achieve the desired outcomes during their training.

counseling More of the attention is devoted to clarifying, deconstructing, and resolving problems than brainstorming around optimal goals and paths toward goal attainment.

critical incidents Incidents or experiences that have a significant impact on one's life and thinking.

curiosity The desire to know and understand. A powerful intrinsic motivator for learning, behavior, creativity, and growth.

D

deliberate practice Foundation by which novices become experts. Focuses primarily on the cultivation of expertise, which is founded on the belief that experts are created through repeated and deliberate practice over an extensive length of time.

distributive justice Rewards appropriate for effort.

diversity The representation of different people within an organization.

dual process theory Adapted from the psychology literature to help explain the ways in which clinicians arrive at medical decisions. Decisions are made via two cognitive pathways called system 1 (thinking fast) and system 2 (thinking slow).

E

emotional intelligence The ability to understand and regulate one's own emotions, understand others' emotions, react to both in a productive way, use these skills to make good judgments, and avoid or solve problems.

equality Quality or state of being equal.

equity Justice according to natural law or right, specifically freedom from bias or favoritism.

evaluation matrix Tool for keeping track of the methods considered for collecting data. In its simplest form, a matrix displays evaluation questions in alignment with the data collection strategies that will be used to answer them.

F

faculty development Professional development for educators.

G

general needs assessment Step in curriculum development to determine the gap between the current state and the ideal state.

generative moment An energetic, creative conversation, described as relational flow or the intuitive dance, where a coach helps coachees explore new ideas and vantage points freely until they experience a small shift in learning, insight, perspective, or attitude that perceptibly increases their confidence in overcoming a challenge.

generous listening Being fully attentive to the person speaking.

goal-based evaluation Determines the extent to which a program has achieved its goals.

group coaching   A coach trained in group coaching techniques provides coaching to a group of coachees together, coaching one coachee at a time and encouraging group members to coach and support each other.

growth mindset   One of the four internal characteristics that drive the Master Adaptive Learner process. It is a positive belief pattern held about one's own intelligence and capacity for learning being open to ongoing improvement. The other three characteristics are motivation, curiosity, and resilience.

GROW tool   A four-step inquiry. Stands for goal, reality, options, and way forward.

H

hope psychology   A theory developed by Charles Snyder. One part of the theory asserts that hope (and confidence) increase when people have generated at least three new ideas or strategies to address a challenge, giving them more hope that they have the creative ability to identify more strategies if the first three don't succeed.

I

immunity to change   An advanced form of cognitive behavioral coaching. Based on the subject-object theory in adult development, which in brief is the simple mechanism by which adults develop maturity through processing life experiences, moving elements in their minds from subject to object.

imposter syndrome   Doubting one's abilities and feeling like a fraud. Frequently inaccurate.

inclusion   Ensuring everyone has an equal opportunity to contribute to and influence every part and level of an institution.

individual coaching   Coachees speak to the coach directly, one-on-one, whether it's a phone call, video-conferencing, or an in-person session. Private and confidential.

inequity   An injustice or unfairness.

informed self-assessment   Use of external information to inform and generate a more accurate concept of the individual's knowledge, skills, and attitudes.

instructional designer   An expert who understands how to classify outcomes, generate measurable objectives, select appropriate assessment and teaching strategies, and design effective instruction.

intentional change theory   A leadership coaching model developed by Richard Boyatzis and collaborators as a direct application of self-determination theory.

intrinsic motivation   Spontaneous propensity of people to take interest in their inner and outer worlds in an attempt to engage, interact, master, and understand, without needing external rewards.

J

justice   All persons are entitled to access and benefit from the contributions, processes, procedures, and services being conducted.

K

Kern's six steps   Framework for curriculum development in medical education.

Kirkpatrick's model   Used for conducting outcome evaluations of training programs. Has four levels: reaction/satisfaction, learning, behavior, and results.

Kotter's eight-step process   A model for change management.

L

learning environment   The contexts, cultures, and diverse physical locations in which individuals learn, which are all the more complex in health care.

logic model   A program planning tool to help with program design.

M

master adaptive learner   A learner who uses a metacognitive approach to self-regulated learning that leads to the development and demonstration of adaptive expertise.

mentoring   Mentors often have in-depth personal knowledge of their learners. Assumes a more intimate relationship. The mentor feels personal responsibility and, in turn, fulfillment when the protégé succeeds. Not to be confused with coaching or advising.

milestones   Knowledge, skills, attitudes, and other attributes for each of the Accreditation Council for Graduate Medical Education competencies that describe the development of competence from an early learner up to and beyond that expected for unsupervised practice.

mindfulness   Awareness that arises through paying attention, on purpose, in the present moment, nonjudgmentally, in the service of self-understanding and wisdom. The coaching process often helps coachees become more mindful.

motivational interviewing   An evidence-based theory centered on conversational techniques that engage a coachee's sense of autonomy, curiosity, motivation, competence, and creativity.

Myers-Briggs type indicator   An introspective self-report questionnaire indicating differing psychological preferences in how people perceive the world and make decisions.

N

near-peer coaching   A dyadic platonic relationship between a more experienced student (coach) and a less experienced student (coachee) at the same institution, with frequent, direct, face-to-face contact.

nonviolent communication   A widely used tool in coaching that has four steps for efficiently processing and learning from emotions.

O

observed standardized clinical exams (OSCEs)   A versatile multipurpose evaluative tool that can be used to evaluate health care professionals in a clinical setting and assess competency based on objective testing through direct observation.

outcomes-based evaluation   Measures the actual impacts of the coaching program itself.

P

peer-assessment debriefing instrument   A self and peer assessment designed to measure a debriefers' effectiveness. Grounded in current scientific debriefing literature and peer review methodology.

peer coaching   Confidential, nonevaluative process through which two or more colleagues work together to improve each other.

performance coaching   Series of techniques aiming to bring about continuous improvement in an individual's performance.

positive emotions   Vital resources for navigating self-change and improving well-being.

positive psychology The scientific study of what makes life most worth living, focusing on both individual and societal well-being.

positive psychology coaching Approach to coaching that focuses on strengths and emphasizes engagement, meaning, and accomplishment.

prejudice A preconceived opinion about a person or group without actual logic or experience.

primary psychological needs Comprised of autonomy, competence, and relatedness, which are preconditions for well-being and autonomous self-regulation of behavior and growth.

privilege Right or immunity granted as a particular benefit, advantage, or favor.

process-based evaluation Focuses on a program's activities rather than its outcomes and offers insight into the program's implementation and management.

professional development Learning to earn or maintain professional credentials such as academic degrees to formal coursework, attending conferences, and informal learning opportunities situated in practice. Intensive and collaborative, ideally incorporating an evaluative stage.

professional identity formation The process of internalizing a profession's core values and beliefs.

psychological capital Evidence-based resources that support resilience, positive change, well-being, and positive organizational cultures.

psychological flexibility The ability to be fully conscious, embrace emotional experiences, and be guided in actions by heartfelt values.

psychological safety When the coachee feels safe to authentically share their values, experiences, perspectives, and concerns with the coach and feels safe to explore difficult topics such as feedback, conflicts, or equity and inclusion issues.

R

R2C2 framework A framework for feedback conversations that emphasize relationships and performance improvement. Stands for relationship, reaction, content, and coaching.

racism Prejudice, discrimination, or antagonism directed against a person or people on the basis of their membership in a particular minoritized or marginalized racial or ethnic group.

reflective practice Habit of reflecting on one's actions for the purpose of continuous learning.

resilience Capacity to recover quickly from difficulties.

return on investment A measurement to show a return on learning, development, and performance improvement costs for an organization.

S

self-compassion Extending compassion to oneself in instances of perceived inadequacy, failure, or general suffering.

self-determination theory A macro theory of human motivation and personality that concerns people's inherent growth tendencies and innate psychological needs. It is concerned with the motivation behind choices people make without external influence and interference.

self-directed learning A process by which individuals take the initiative, with or without the assistance of others, in diagnosing their learning needs, formulating learning goals, identifying human and material resources for learning, and choosing and implementing appropriate learning.

self-efficacy Personal judgment of how well or poorly a person is able to cope with a given situation, or perform a specific task or activity, based on the skills they have and the circumstances they face.

self-insight The clarity of one's understanding of one's thoughts, feelings, and behavior. A metacognitive factor central to the process of purposeful, directed change and meaning making.

SMART goals An acronym that stands for specific, measurable, achievable, relevant, and time-based.

socialization The process by which an individual learns how to be a member of a group.

stereotype Oversimplified image of a group based on beliefs that may or may not be entirely true.

subject-object theory The simple mechanism by which adults develop maturity through processing life experiences, moving elements in their minds from subject to object.

SWOT A strategic planning technique used to help a person or organization identify strengths, weaknesses, opportunities, and threats.

T

targeted needs assessment A step in curriculum development to determine the needs of a specific group of learners to inform curricular goals, objectives, and educational strategies.

Thomas-Kilmann Conflict Mode Instrument A tool developed to measure an individual's response to conflict situations.

U

unconditional regard Means that coaches accept and value coachees without conditions or contingents, which supports and satisfies coachees' autonomy needs.

underrepresented in medicine (UiM) Demographic populations that are underrepresented in the medical profession relative to their numbers in the general population.

V

VIA Inventory of Strengths (VIA-IS) A proprietary psychological assessment measure designed to identify an individual's profile of character strengths. Formerly known as the Values in Action Inventory.

W

WOOP behavior change tool Stands for wish, outcome, obstacle, plan. Ensures that goals aren't clarified until the first three steps are complete and that goals are focused on overcoming obstacles and increasing confidence.

INDEX

Page numbers followed by *f* indicate figures; *b*, boxes; *t*, tables.